Atlas of Surgical Approaches
in Small Animal
ORTHOPAEDICS

Title:

Atlas of Surgical Approaches in Small Animal Orthopaedics.
Thoracic and Pelvic Limbs

Authors:

Jordi Franch DVM PhD
Associate Professor of Orthopaedic Surgery
Veterinary School
Autonomous University of Barcelona. Spain

Carlos López DVM PhD
Associate Professor of Anatomy and Embryology
Veterinary School
Autonomous University of Barcelona. Spain

Translation:

Guillem Riera, DVM
Judith Fulls, VN

Revision of the translated version:

Jordi Franch DVM PhD
Carlos López DVM PhD
Ronan Fitzgerald, BVetMed.,MRCVS,
Bayer Animal Health, UK

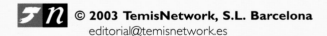 **© 2003 TemisNetwork, S.L. Barcelona**
editorial@temisnetwork.es

I.S.B.N.: 84-95492-23-7

Atlas of Surgical Approaches
in *Small Animal*
ORTHOPAEDICS

Jordi Franch DVM PhD
Associate Professor of Orthopaedic Surgery
Veterinary School
Autonomous University of Barcelona. Spain

Carlos López DVM PhD
Associate Professor of Anatomy and Embryology
Veterinary School
Autonomous University of Barcelona. Spain

𝑛

TemisNetwork S.L.

"For a bone is a plant, with its roots in the soft tissues, and when its vascular connections are damaged, it often requires, not the technique of a cabinet maker, but the patient care and understanding of a gardener."

Girdlstone, 1932

preface

In 1991, DL Piermattei was explaining to one of the authors his hobby of flying his aeroplane over the Rocky Mountains. His passion for flying and seeing the world from an aerial perspective, probably made him realise something that many of us ignore; namely, that the best approach to a bone is not always the most straightforward. In the field of veterinary orthopaedics, the name of Piermattei is synonymous with surgical approaches. Without detracting from other publications in this field, his book 'An Atlas of Surgical Approaches to the Bones and Joints of the Dog and Cat' represents the gold standard. From the first edition, which was published in 1966, to the third (and most recent) in 1993, his work is constantly referred to, in any book or publication dealing with veterinary orthopaedics. Many veterinary surgeons have been grateful for the invaluable assistance provided by this book, when confronted by an orthopaedic procedure.

Our intention with this new publication is not to challenge the position occupied by Professor Piermattei's book, but to complement it. The pictures of the different stages of a surgical approach, together with the accompanying illustrations and descriptions, should offer an accurate and useful guide for the surgeon.

Our objective with this book is to describe a selection of surgical approaches frequently used in small animal orthopaedic surgery; it is not however our intention to exhaustively document all existing approaches. It is of course the case that an individual surgeon may choose alternatives which may have been published elsewhere and not described in this book, or perhaps perform his or her own modifications, based on personal experience.

In order to make the pictures as relevant as possible to the surgeon, we have not used cadavers which were preserved in formaldehyde. It is our belief that this decision lends more weight to the dissection, despite the inevitable and progressive deterioration of the anatomical structures. The reader will notice the variation in the size and shape of the limbs used, despite our efforts to ensure homogeneity. This is because the animals used in our work all died from other causes and were not put down in order to provide specimens for this book.

By the same token, it is sometimes difficult to carry out an approach as we would in a clinical situation and see, at the same time, all of the relevant anatomical structures. For this reason, the areas of exposure shown in this atlas are wider than would be the case during surgery. In some instances we have removed the subcutaneous fat, fascia etc. Closure of the operation site is performed routinely and only in some specific instances, is the closure described in the book.

Whenever possible, structures are named according to the Nomina Anatomica Veterinaria; only in certain cases have we used names which are in common use in orthopaedics, but which are not listed in the NAV.

We hope that this atlas will be of use, both to the student and the experienced surgeon, and that it represents a worthwhile addition to the body of literature relating to veterinary orthopaedics.

We are very grateful to all the people who believed in this project and helped to make it possible. We would like to mention the excellent work of Lidia Di Blasi in the illustrations, the patience and professionalism of Ascen Álvarez in the graphic design and the support of TemisNetwork and Bayer.

We would like to dedicate our work to Olga, Roger, Eva, Pau and Enric from whom so many family hours have been stolen to produce this book.

THE AUTHORS

Abbreviations:

A., Aa.	- Artery, arteries		**N., Nn.**	- Nerve, nerves
V., Vv.	- Vein, veins		**P.**	- Part
M., Mm.	- Muscle, muscles			

contents

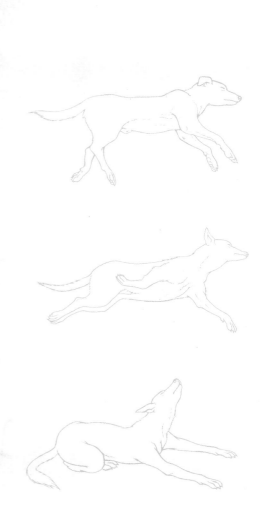

THORACIC

Limb

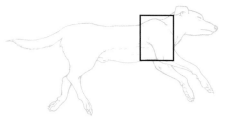
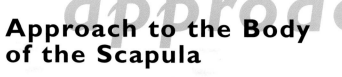
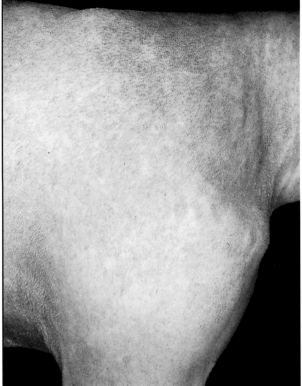

fig.1.1

The animal is in left lateral recumbency. Lateral view of the right thoracic limb.

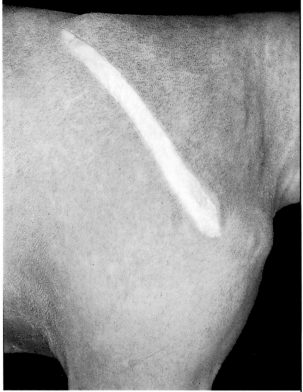

fig.1.2

The cutaneous incision is performed over the spine of the scapula and extended depending on the area of interest.

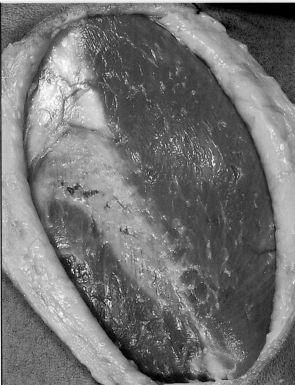

fig.1.3

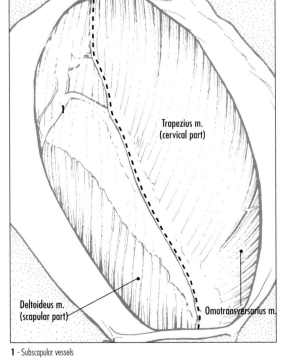

Trapezius m.
(cervical part)

Deltoideus m.
(scapular part)

Omotransversarius m.

1 - Subscapular vessels

Once the skin and fascia have been dissected, an incision is made over the insertion of the deltoideus (scapular part), omotransversarius and trapezius (cervical part) muscles, along the spine.

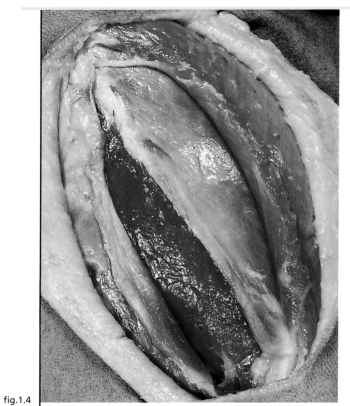

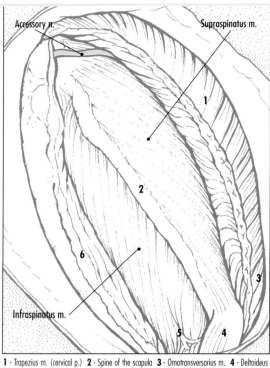

1 - Trapezius m. (cervical p.) **2** - Spine of the scapula **3** - Omotransversarius m. **4** - Deltoideus m. (acromial p.) **5** - Caudal circumflex humeral vessels **6** - Deltoideus m. (scapular p.)

fig.1.4

Cranial retraction of the omotransversarius and trapezius muscles, and caudal retraction of the scapular portion of the deltoideus muscle, allows us to recognise the supraspinatus and infraspinatus muscles. Detachment of the proximal portion of the trapezius muscle (cervical part) must be done carefully to avoid damaging the accessory nerve.

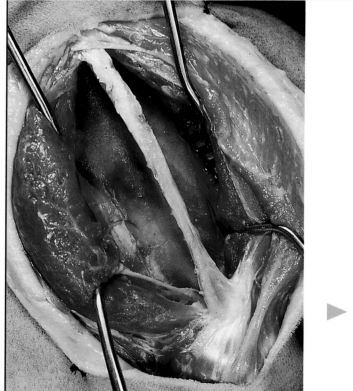

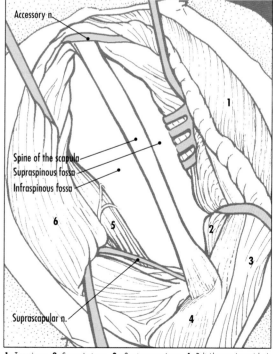

1 - Trapezius m. **2** - Supraspinatus m. **3** - Omotransversarius m. **4** - Deltoideus m. (acromial p.) **5** - Teres minor m. **6** - Infraspinatus m.

fig.1.5

Elevation of the infraspinatus and supraspinatus exposes the spine and body of the scapula.

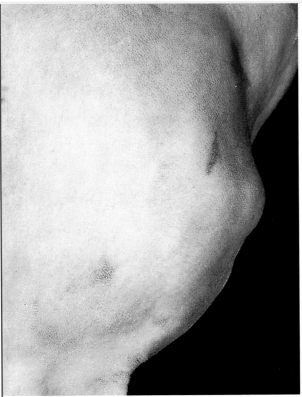

fig.2.1

The animal is in left lateral recumbency. Lateral view of the right thoracic limb.

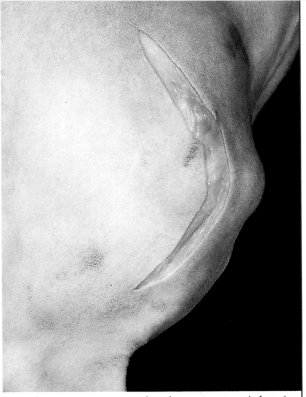

fig.2.2

A curved cutaneous incision, centred on the acromion, extends from the middle of the scapular spine, over the lateral aspect of the humerus, to the midpoint of the humeral diaphysis.

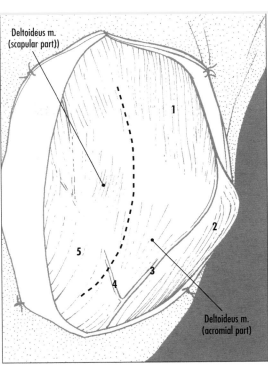

Deltoideus m.
(scapular part))

Deltoideus m.
(acromial part)

1 - Omotransversarius m. **2** - Brachiocephalicus m. **3** - Omobrachial v. **4** - Axillobrachial v.
5 - Triceps brachii m.

fig.2.3

Skin and subcutaneous tissue retraction allows recognition of the fascia, which will be incised in the same fashion.

2

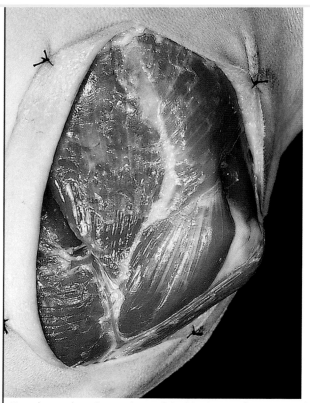

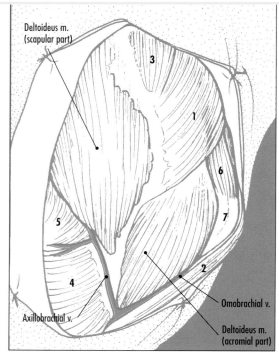

1 - Omotransversarius m. 2 - Brachiocephalicus m. 3 - Trapezius m. (cervical p.) 4 - Triceps brachii m. (lateral head) 5 - Triceps brachii m. (long head) 6 - Supraspinatus m. 7 - Greater tubercle of the humerus

fig.2.4

Next, the scapular and acromial parts of the deltoideus muscle are separated. The picture is taken after the majority of the deep fascia has been removed to help the reader visualise the structures.

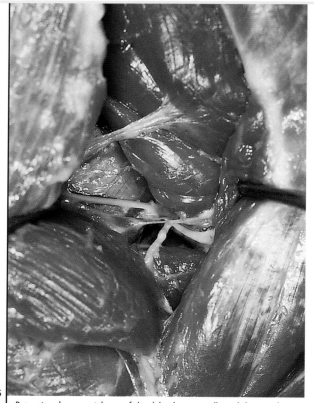

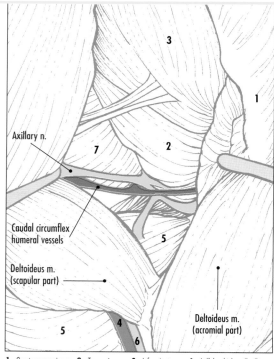

1 - Omotransversarius m. 2 - Teres minor m. 3 - Infraspinatus m. 4 - Axillobrachial v. 5 - Triceps brachii m. (lateral head) 6 - Cranial lateral cutaneous brachial n. 7 - Triceps brachii m. (long head)

fig.2.5

Retracting the acromial part of the deltoideus cranially and the spinal part caudally, the axillary nerve and the caudal circumflex humeral vessels are identified.

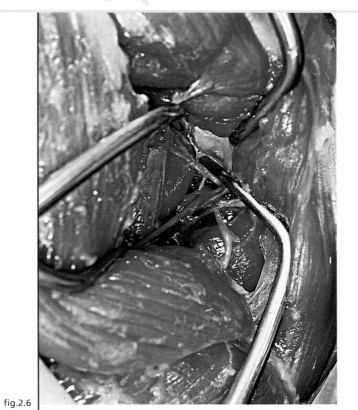

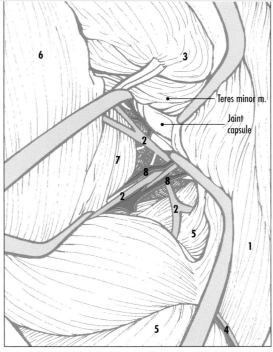

Joint location is helped by moving the limb at the same time as palpation deep and caudal to the teres minor muscle is performed.

Teres minor m.

Joint capsule

1 - Deltoideus m. (acromial p.) **2** - Axillary n. **3** - Infraspinatus m. **4** - Axillobrachial v., cranial lateral cutaneous brachial n. **5** - Triceps brachii m. (lateral head) **6** - Deltoideus m. (scapular p.)
7 - Triceps brachii m. (long head) **8** - Caudal circumflex humeral vessels

fig.2.6

The articular capsule of the shoulder joint is exposed by cranial retraction of the teres minor muscle.

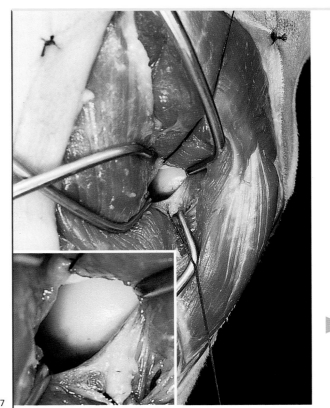

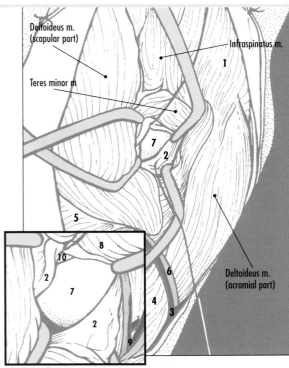

Deltoideus m. (scapular part)

Infraspinatus m.

Teres minor m

Deltoideus m. (acromial part)

Improving the access to the articular surfaces is achieved by accessing the joint between the teres minor and infraspinatus muscles or by severing the insertion of the infraspinatus muscle close to the base of the greater tubercle.

1 - Omotransversarius m. **2** - Joint capsule **3** - Axillobrachial v. **4** - Triceps brachii m. (lateral head)
5 - Triceps brachii m. (long head) **6** - Cranial lateral cutaneous brachial n. **7** - Humeral head **8** -
Teres minor m. **9** - Axillary n., caudal circumflex humeral vessels. **10** - Glenoid rim

fig.2.7

Incision of the joint capsule exposes the caudal aspect of the shoulder joint. Most of the head of the humerus can be seen by adducting and internally rotating the humerus.

OSTEOTOMY OF THE ACROMION

2

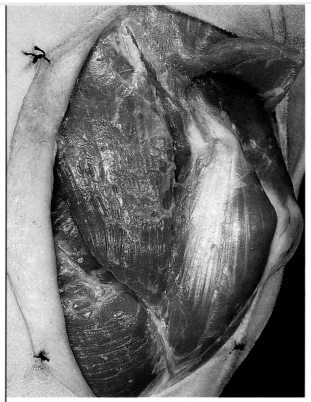

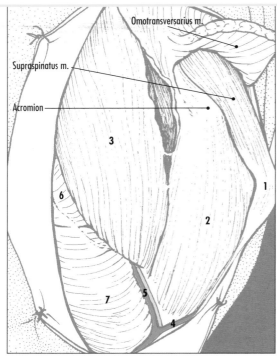

1 - Greater tubercle of the humerus **2** - Deltoideus m. (acromial p.) **3** - Deltoideus m. (scapular p.) **4** - Omobrachial v. **5** - Axillobrachial v.; cranial lateral cutaneous brachial n. **6** - Triceps brachii m. (long head) **7** - Triceps brachii m. (lateral head)

fig.2.8

The approach to the shoulder by osteotomy of the acromion follows the same initial steps of the above approach (see fig. 2.1, 2.2, 2.3 and 2.4). The omotransversarius muscle is incised and retracted cranially to expose the acromion.

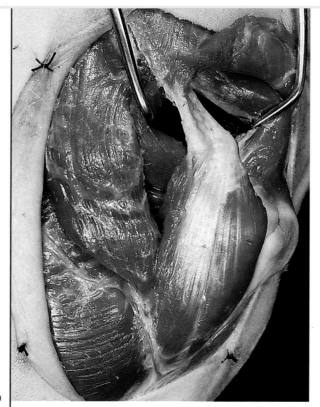

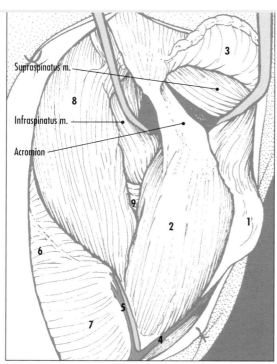

1 - Greater tubercle of the humerus **2** - Deltoideus m. (acromial p.) **3** - Omotransversarius m. **4** - Omobrachial v. **5** - Axillobrachial v. ; cranial lateral cutaneous brachial n. **6** - Triceps brachii m. (long head) **7** - Triceps brachii m. (lateral head) **8** - Deltoideus m. (scapular p.) **9** - Teres minor m.

fig.2.9

The base of the acromion is exposed by separation of the supraspinatus muscle cranially and the infraspinatus muscle caudally.

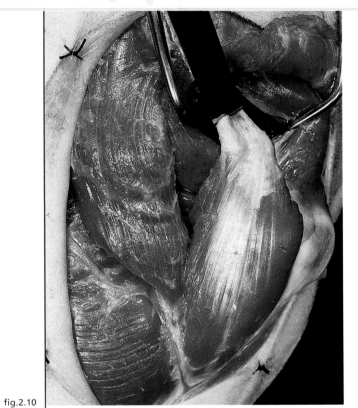

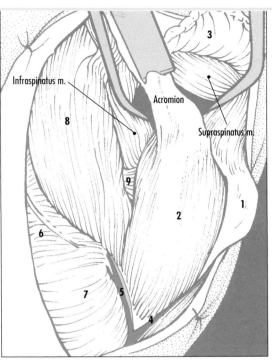

The osteotomized acromion is fixed by a tension band device or crossed cerclages.

Infraspinatus m.

Acromion

Supraspinatus m.

1 - Greater tubercle of the humerus **2** - Deltoideus m. (acromial p.) **3** - Omotransversarius m. **4** - Omobrachial v. **5** - Axillobrachial v. ; cranial lateral cutaneous brachial n. **6** - Triceps brachii m. (long head) **7** - Triceps brachii m. (lateral head) **8** - Deltoideus m. (scapular p.) **9** - Teres minor m.

fig.2.10

The osteotomy is performed using a chisel. The angle of the chisel is such that it involves most of the acromion without affecting the base of the scapular spine, in order to avoid injuring the suprascapular nerve (see fig.2.11).

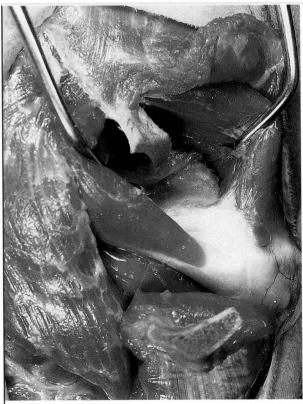

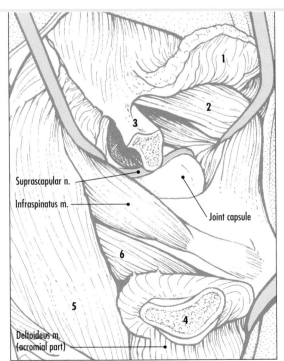

Suprascapular n.

Infraspinatus m.

Joint capsule

Deltoideus m. (acromial part)

1 - Omotransversarius m. **2** - Supraspinatus m. **3** - Spine of the scapula **4** - Acromion **5** - Deltoideus m. (scapular p.) **6** - Teres minor m.

fig.2.11

Once the osteotomy has been performed, the acromial part of the deltoideus muscle is retracted distally, exposing the articular capsule underneath.

2

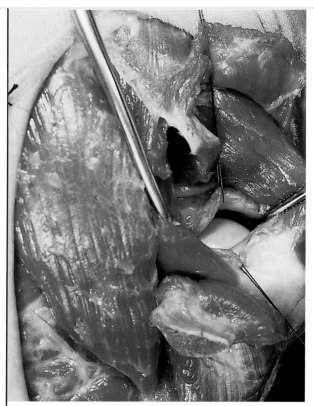

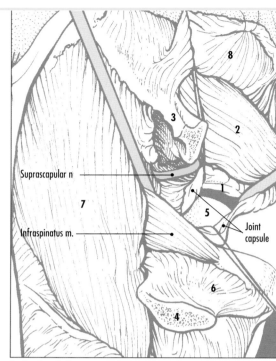

1 - Glenoid rim 2 - Supraspinatus m. 3 - Spine of the scapula 4 - Detached acromion
5 - Humeral head 6 - Deltoideus m. (acromial p.) 7 - Deltoideus m. (scapular p.)
8 - Omotransversarius m.

fig.2.12

The incision to the joint capsule allows visualization of the lateral aspect of the shoulder joint.

In very small or young dogs and cats, tenotomy of the acromial portion of the deltoideus muscle is preferred over osteotomy. The tendon is sutured back using bone tunnels created in the acromion.

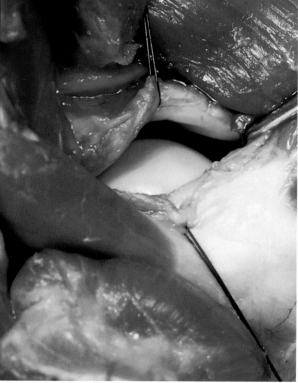

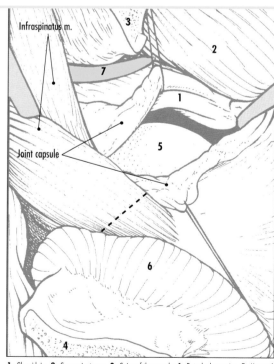

1 - Glenoid rim 2 - Supraspinatus m. 3 - Spine of the scapula 4 - Detached acromion 5 - Humeral head 6 - Deltoideus m. (acromial part) 7 - Suprascapular n.

fig.2.13

Enlarged view of the picture 2.12. Partial or total tenotomy of the infraspinatus muscle (dotted line) improves the approach caudally.

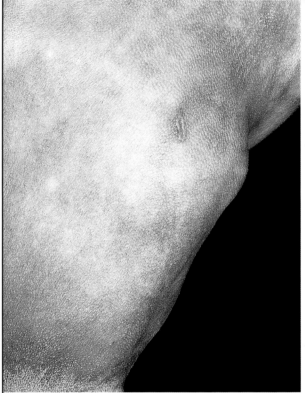

fig.2.14

The animal is in left lateral recumbency. Lateral view of the right thoracic limb.

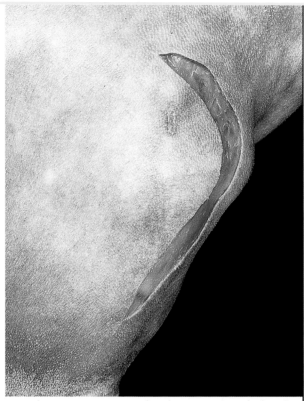

fig.2.15

A curved cutaneous incision, centred on the acromion, extends along the distal half of the scapular spine, over the lateral aspect of the humerus, to the midpoint of the humeral diaphysis.

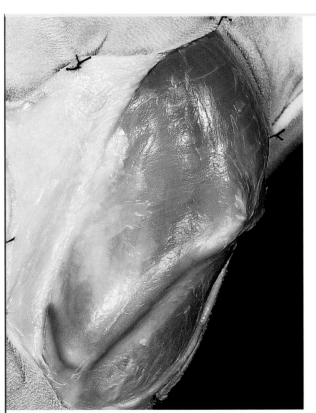

fig.2.16

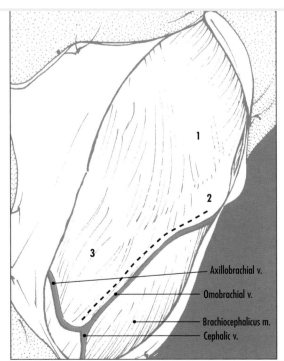

Axillobrachial v.

Omobrachial v.

Brachiocephalicus m.

Cephalic v.

1 - Omotransversarius m. **2** - Greater tubercle of the humerus **3** - Deltoideus m. (acromial p.)

Skin and subcutaneous tissue retraction allows visualisation of the fascia that will be incised, following the caudolateral edge of the brachiocephalicus muscle.

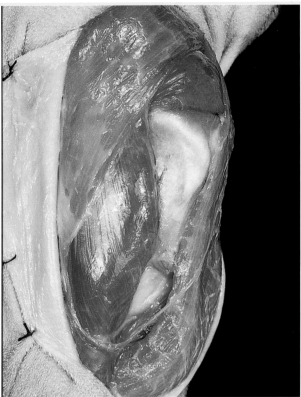

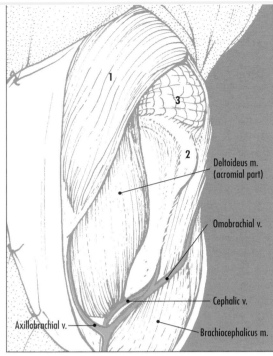

1 - Omotransversarius m.   2 - Greater tubercle of the humerus   3 - Supraspinatus m.

fig.2.17

The photo shows the area of interest after the majority of the deep fascia has been removed.

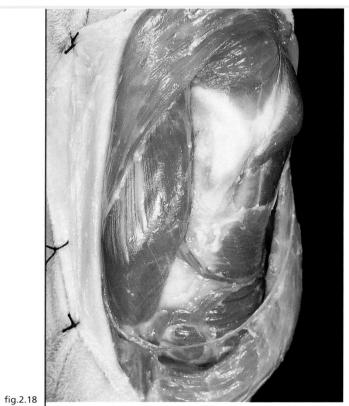

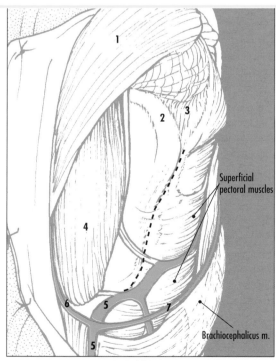

1 - Omotransversarius m.   2 - Greater tubercle of the humerus   3 - Supraspinatus m.   4 - Deltoideus m. (acromial p.)   5 - Cephalic v.   6 - Axillobrachial v.   7 - Omobrachial v.

fig.2.18

After craniomedial retraction of the brachiocephalicus muscle, an incision is made at the humeral insertion of the superficial pectoral muscles.

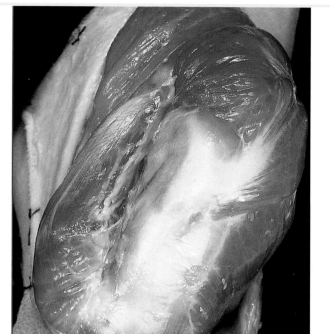

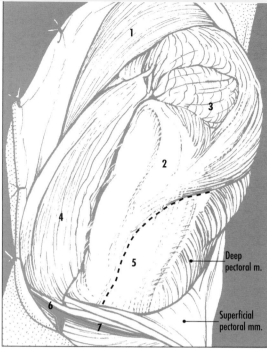

Closure is performed by suturing the superficial and deep pectoral muscles to the acromial portion of the deltoideus muscle.

1 - Omotransversarius m. **2** - Greater tubercle of the humerus **3** - Supraspinatus m. **4** - Deltoideus m. (acromial p.) **5** - Biceps brachii m. **6** - Axillobrachial v. **7** - Omobrachial v.

fig.2.19

Cranial view of the shoulder. Caudoventral reflection of the superficial pectoral muscles, exposes the insertion of the deep pectoral muscle that will be incised.

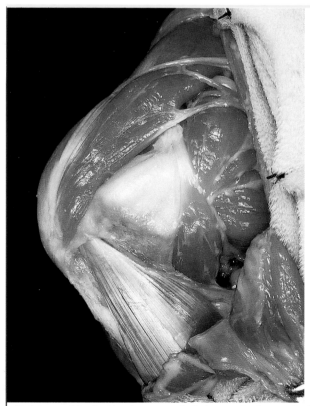

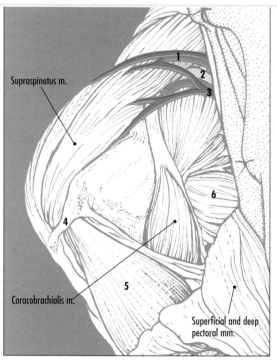

1 - Acromial branch of the superficial cervical a. and v. **2** - Suprascapular n. **3** - Suprascapular a. and v. **4** - Transverse humeral ligament **5** - Biceps brachii m. **6** - Subscapularis m.

fig.2.20

Medial view of the shoulder after rotating the limb externally. The superficial and deep pectoral muscles have been retracted ventrally and medially. In order to help the identification of the structures, the approach has been enlarged medially in this photo.

OSTEOTOMY OF THE GREATER TUBERCLE

2

The osteotomized greater tubercle is reattached with a tension band wire, two lag screws or two Kirschner wires, inserted perpendicular to each plane of the osteotomy.

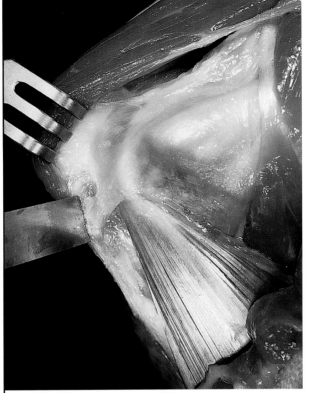

fig.2.21

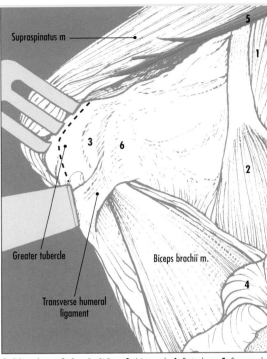

Supraspinatus m

Greater tubercle

Transverse humeral ligament

Biceps brachii m.

1 - Subscapularis m. **2** - Coracobrachialis m. **3** - Joint capsule **4** - Pectoral mm. **5** - Suprascapular vessels **6** - Lesser tubercle of the humerus

Osteotomy of the greater tubercle should be performed on the medial aspect and follow the two planes illustrated. It will affect the insertion of the tendon of the supraspinatus muscle but should not involve the cranial insertion of the transverse humeral ligament.

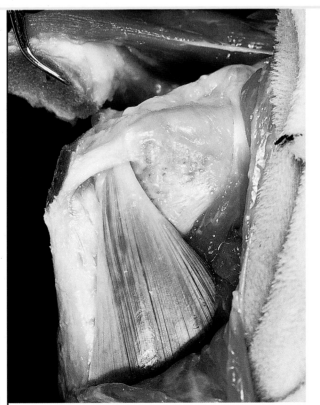

fig.2.22

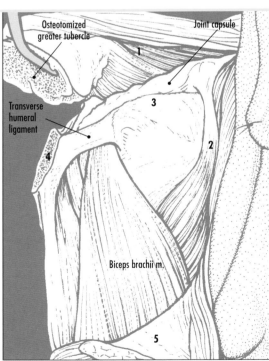

Osteotomized greater tubercle

Joint capsule

Transverse humeral ligament

Biceps brachii m.

1 - Supraspinatus m. **2** - Coracobrachialis m. **3** - Lesser tubercle of the humerus **4** - Greater tubercle of the humerus **5** - Pectoral mm.

Once the osteotomy has been performed, the supraspinatus muscle and the separated portion of the greater tubercle are reflected dorsally.

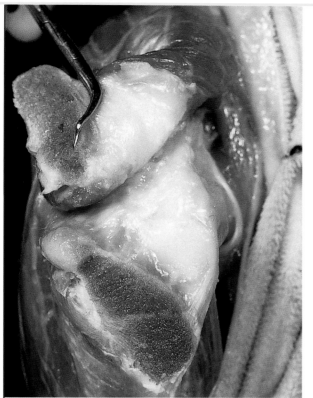

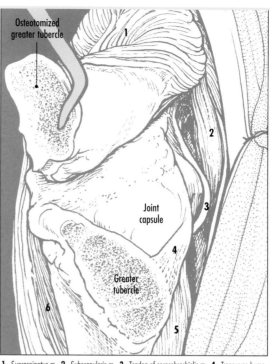

1 - Supraspinatus m. **2** - Subscapularis m. **3** - Tendon of coracobrachialis m. **4** - Transverse humeral ligament **5** - Biceps brachii m. **6** - Deltoideus m. (acromial p.)

fig.2.23

Cranial view of the shoulder. Dorsal retraction of the greater tubercle allows the visualisation of the joint capsule.

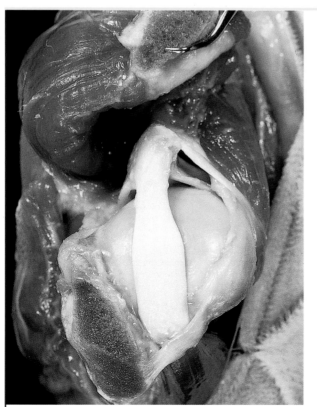

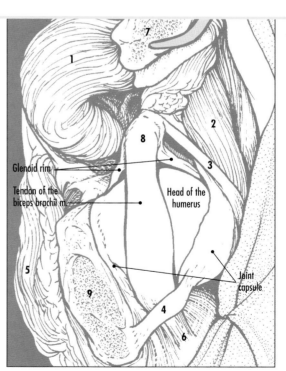

1 - Supraspinatus m. **2** - Subscapularis m. **3** - Tendon of coracobrachialis m. **4** - Transverse humeral ligament **5** - Deltoideus m. (acromial p.) **6** - Biceps brachii m. **7** - Osteotomized greater tubercle **8** - Supraglenoid tubercle of the scapula **9** - Greater tubercle

fig.2.24

Arthrotomy is performed parallel to the biceps brachii tendon (intra-articular, but palpable) to access the shoulder joint. In this picture the articular capsule has been removed.

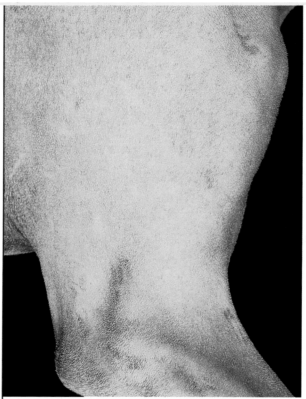

fig.3.1

The animal is in left lateral recumbency. Lateral view of the right thoracic limb.

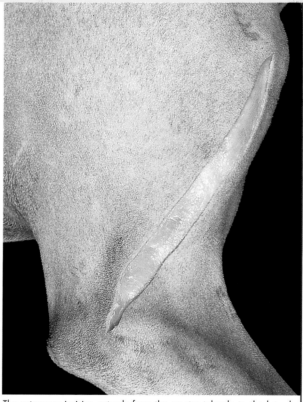

fig.3.2

The cutaneous incision extends from the greater tubercle to the lateral epicondyle in order to expose the whole bone. The incision follows the craniolateral edge of the humerus.

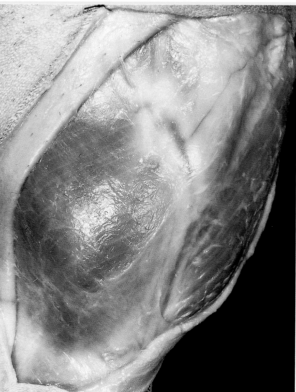

Triceps brachii m.
(lateral head)

Brachiocephalicus m.

1 - Omobrachial v. **2** - Axillobrachial v. **3** - Cephalic v.

fig.3.3

Once the skin and subcutaneous tissues are retracted, the deep fascia is incised along the lateral border of the brachiocephalicus muscle, and ends close to the axillobrachial vein. Distal to this point the fascia is incised following the cranial border of the lateral head of the triceps brachii muscle, avoiding the branches of the radial nerve which are deep to it (see fig.3.4).

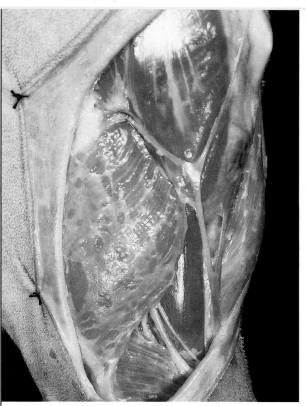

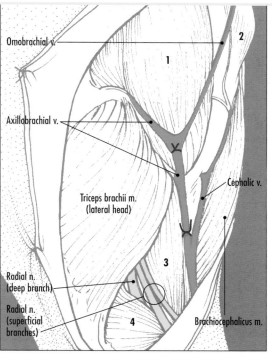

Omobrachial v.

2

1

Axillobrachial v.

Cephalic v.

Triceps brachii m.
(lateral head)

Radial n.
(deep branch)

Radial n.
(superficial
branches)

3

4

Brachiocephalicus m.

1 - Deltoideus m. (acromial p.) **2** - Greater tubercle of the humerus **3** - Brachialis m. **4** - Extensor carpi radialis m.

fig.3.4

In order to facilitate the visualisation of the anatomical structures, the deep fascia has been removed. The axillobrachial vein, located between the cephalic and omobrachial veins, is isolated prior to ligation.

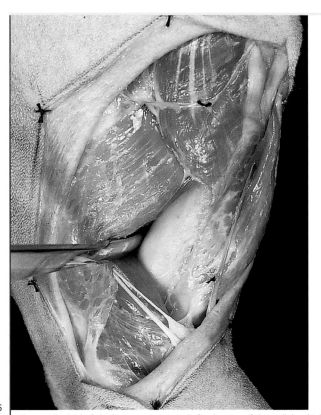

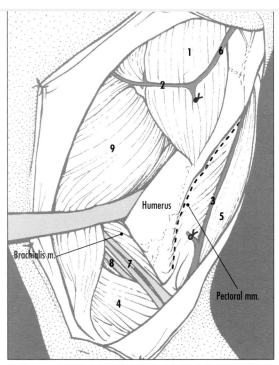

1   6

2

9

Humerus

3

5

Brachialis m.

8   7

Pectoral mm.

4

1 - Deltoideus m. (acromial p.) **2** - Axillobrachial v. **3** - Cephalic v. **4** - Extensor carpi radialis m. **5** - Brachiocephalicus m. **6** - Omobrachial v. **7** - Superficial branches of radial n. **8** - Deep branch of radial n. **9** - Triceps brachii m. (lateral head)

fig.3.5

The middle third of the humerus is exposed after ligation of the axillobrachial vein and caudal retraction of the brachialis muscle. The approach is enlarged proximally by incising the periosteal insertion of the pectoral muscles (dotted line).

3

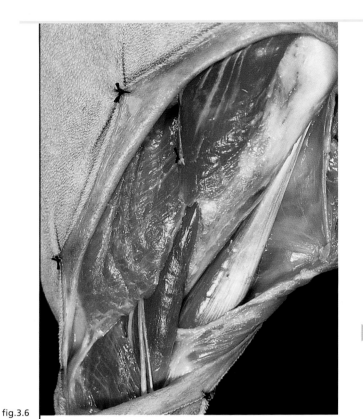

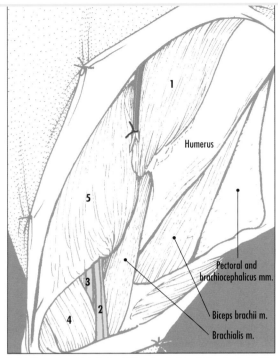

1 - Deltoideus m. (acromial p.) 2 - Superficial branches of radial n. 3 - Deep branch of radial n.
4 - Extensor carpi radialis m. 5 - Triceps brachii m. (lateral head)

fig.3.6

The biceps brachii muscle is exposed by craniomedial retraction of the brachiocephalicus and pectoral muscles.

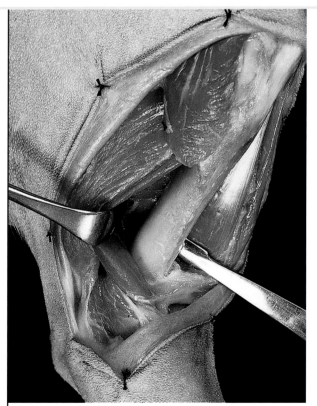

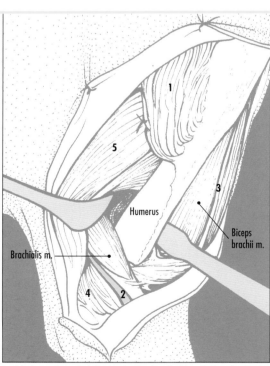

1 - Deltoideus m. (acromial p.) 2 - Superficial branches of radial n. 3 - Pectoral and brachiocephalicus mm. 4 - Extensor carpi radialis m. 5 - Triceps brachii m. (lateral head)

fig.3.7

Most of the shaft is exposed by caudal retraction of the brachialis muscle and medial retraction of the biceps brachii muscle.

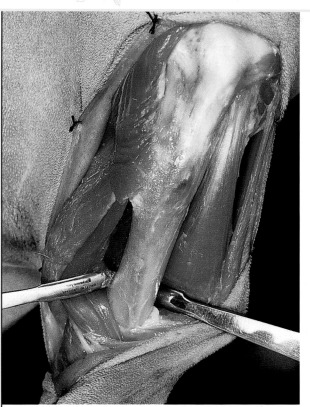

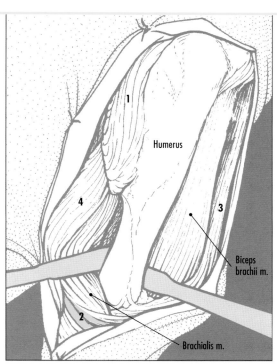

1 - Deltoideus m. (acromial p.) 2 - Superficial branches of radial n. 3 - Pectoral and brachioce-phalicus mm. 4 - Triceps brachii m. (lateral head)

fig.3.8

Cranial view of the brachial area, showing a greater area of exposed bone, facilitating the use of orthopaedic implants.

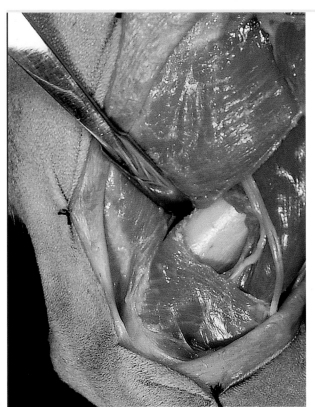

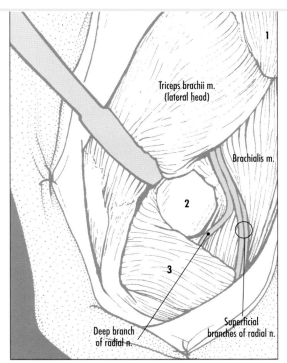

1 - Deltoideus m. 2. Humerus 3. Extensor carpi radialis m.

fig.3.9

Approach to the distal third of the humerus is achieved by caudal retraction of the lateral head of the triceps brachii muscle and cranial retraction of the brachialis muscle together with the branches of the radial nerve. This approach is completed with the lateral approach to the elbow joint as described on page 23.

approach

Medial Approach to the Shaft of the Humerus

4

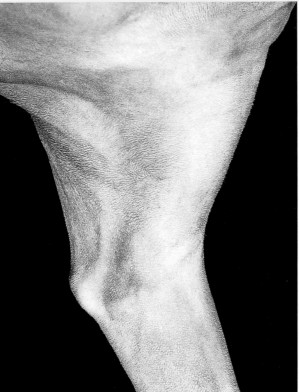

fig.4.1

The animal is in left lateral recumbency. Medial view of the left thoracic limb.

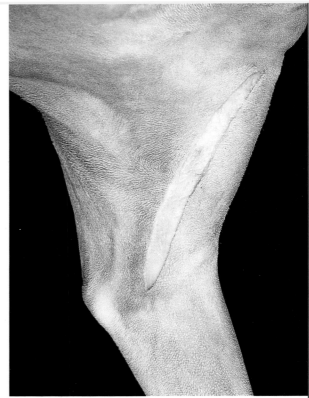

fig.4.2

The cutaneous incision goes from the medial projection of the greater tubercle to the medial humeral epicondyle.

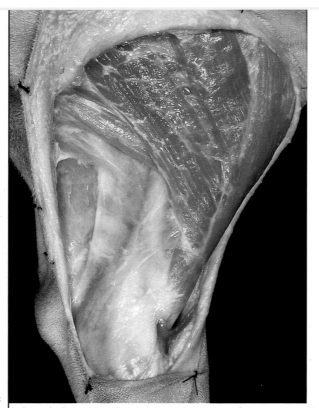

fig.4.3

Skin and subcutaneous tissue are separated in the same fashion. The deep fascia is incised, following the caudal border of the brachiocephalicus muscle. Distally, care must be taken to avoid injuring deeper nerves and blood vessels.

Superficial pectoral mm.

Brachiocephalicus m.

1 - Deep pectoral m. **2** - Biceps brachii m. **3** - Median cubital v. **4** - Superficial brachial v.

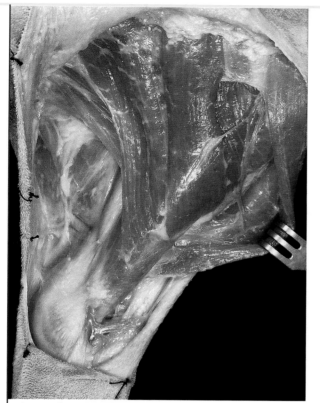

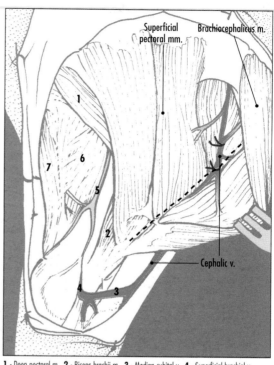

If access is only required to the middle third of the humerus, incision of the pectoral muscles and ligation of the cephalic vein is not necessary.

1 - Deep pectoral m. **2** - Biceps brachii m. **3** - Median cubital v. **4** - Superficial brachial v.
5 - Brachial v. **6** - Triceps brachii m. (long head) **7** - Tensor fasciae antebrachii m.

fig.4.4

After cranially retracting the brachiocephalicus muscle, an incision is made on the insertion of the superficial pectoral muscle. The cephalic vein is located underneath the brachiocephalicus muscle and ligated.

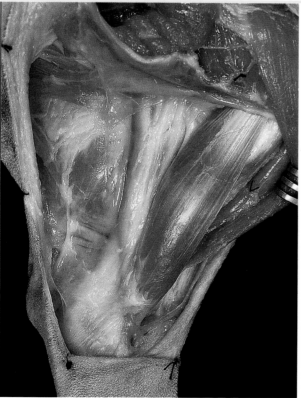

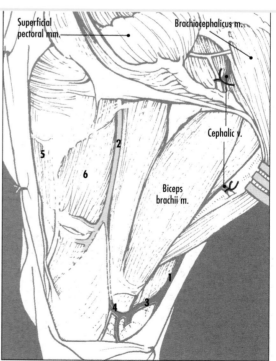

1 - Cephalic v. **2** - Biceps brachii m. **3** - Median cubital v. **4** - Superficial brachial v. **5** - Tensor fasciae antebrachii m. **6** - Triceps brachii m. (long head)

fig.4.5

Biceps brachii muscle, partially covering the humeral shaft, is visualized after retracting the superficial pectoral muscles dorsally.

4

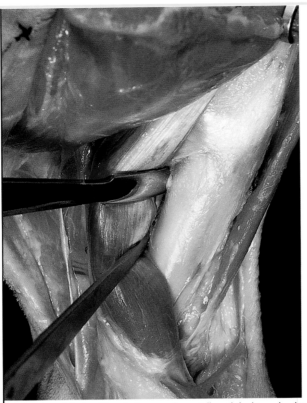

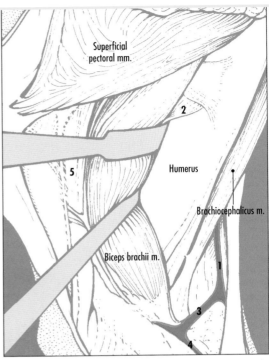

1 - Cephalic v. 2 - Insertion tendons of the teres major and latissimus dorsi mm. 3 - Median cubital v.
4 - Superficial brachial v. 5 - Triceps brachii m. (long head)

fig.4.6

Separation of the brachiocephalicus muscle cranially and the biceps brachii muscle caudally gives access to the proximal two thirds of the medial aspect of the humerus.

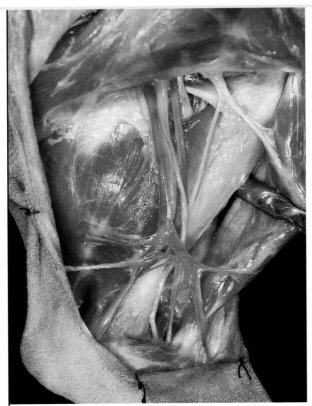

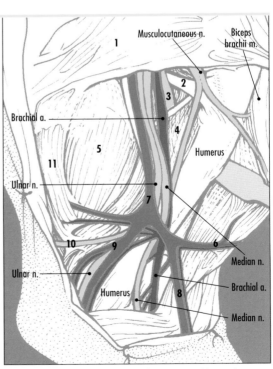

1 - Superficial pectoral mm. 2 - Insertion tendons of the teres major and latissimus dorsi mm.
3 - Radial n. 4 - Triceps brachii m. (medial head) 5 - Triceps brachii m. (long head) 6 - Bicipital
a. and v. 7 - Brachial v. 8 - Superficial brachial a. and v. 9 - Collateral ulnar v. 10 - Caudal cutaneous antebrachial n. 11 - Tensor fasciae antebrachii m.

fig.4.7

Cranial retraction of the biceps brachii muscle is necessary to access the distal third of the medial aspect of the humerus. The important neurovascular structures present at this level must be dissected and retracted in order to reach the medial supracondylar area of the humerus.

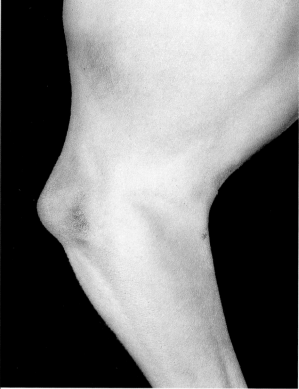

fig.5.1

The animal is in left lateral recumbency. Lateral view of the right thoracic limb.

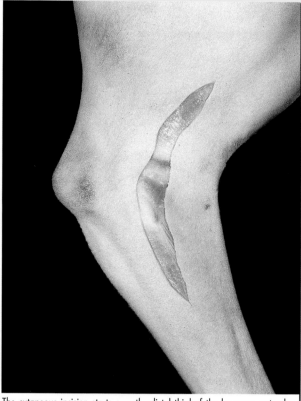

fig.5.2

The cutaneous incision starts over the distal third of the humerus, extends distally over the lateral epicondyle and finishes at the proximal third of the radius.

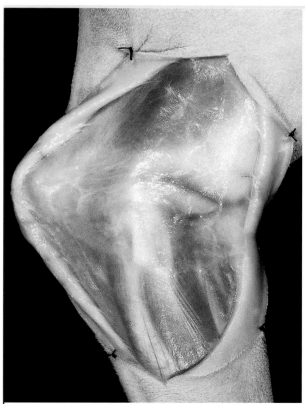

fig.5.3

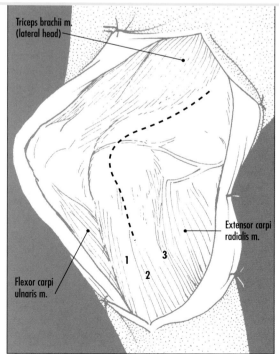

Care must be taken when incising the brachial fascia to avoid damaging the branches of the radial n.

Triceps brachii m. (lateral head)

Extensor carpi radialis m.

Flexor carpi ulnaris m.

1 - Extensor carpi ulnaris m. **2** - Lateral digital extensor m. **3** - Common digital extensor m.

Subcutaneous tissue and superficial fascia are incised and retracted in the same fashion. The deep antebrachial fascia is incised in the same way, while the deep brachial fascia is incised, following the cranial edge of the lateral head of the triceps brachii muscle.

5

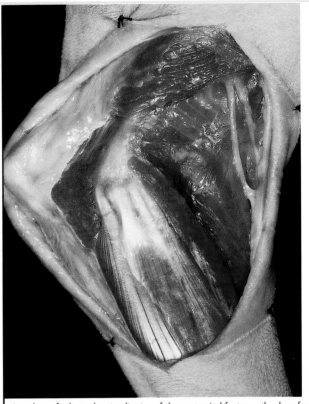

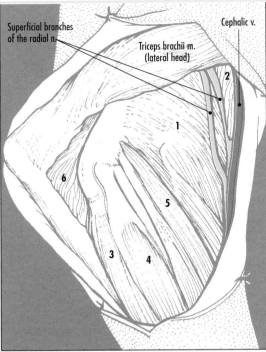

1 - Extensor carpi radialis m. 2 - Brachialis m. 3 - Extensor carpi ulnaris m. 4 - Lateral digital extensor m. 5 - Common digital extensor m. 6 - Anconeus m.

fig.5.4

In order to facilitate the visualisation of the anatomical features, the deep fascia has been removed. It is important to visualise the branches of the radial nerve to avoid any damage during the procedure.

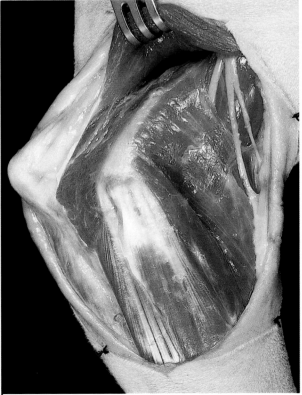

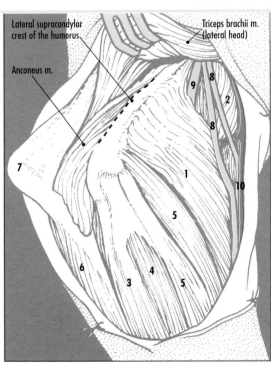

1 - Extensor carpi radialis m. 2 - Brachialis m. 3 - Extensor carpi ulnaris m. 4 - Lateral digital extensor m. 5 - Common digital extensor m. 6 - Flexor carpi ulnaris m. 7 - Olecranon tuberosity 8 - Superficial branches of the radial n. 9 - Deep branch of the radial n. 10 - Cephalic v.

fig.5.5

Proximal retraction of the lateral head of the triceps brachii muscle allows the lateral supracondylar crest to be seen. The next step is the incision of the anconeus muscle´s insertion to that crest (dotted line).

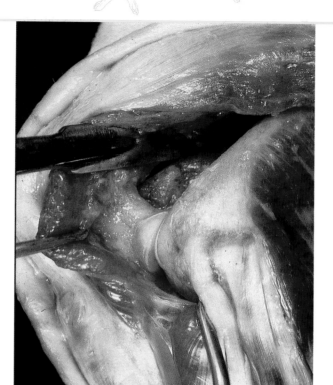

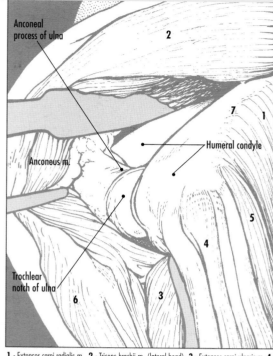

1 - Extensor carpi radialis m. **2** - Triceps brachii m. (lateral head) **3** - Extensor carpi ulnaris m. **4** - Lateral digital extensor m. **5** - Common digital extensor m. **6** - Flexor carpi ulnaris m. **7** - Lateral supracondylar crest of the humerus

fig.5.6

The approach to the humeroulnar joint is completed by caudodorsal retraction of the anconeus muscle.

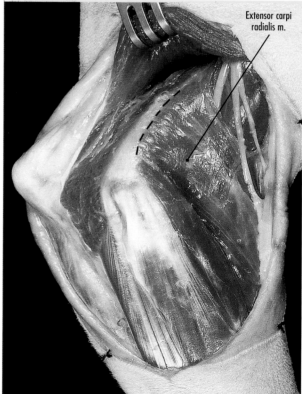

fig.5.7

The cranial compartment of the elbow joint is approached by incising the extensor carpi radialis muscle, on the lateral supracondylar crest. In order to do this, it is necessary to retract the lateral head of the triceps brachii muscle (see fig. 5.5).

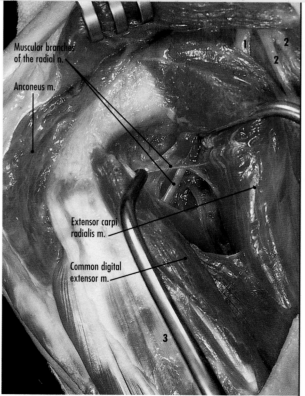

The extensor carpi radialis muscle can be sutured to its insertion, deep fascia or lateral insertion of the anconeus muscle.

fig.5.8

The cranial retraction of the extensor carpi radialis muscle can be improved by dissecting its belly from the common digital extensor muscle.

1 - Deep branch of the radial n. **2**. Superficial branches of the radial n. **3**. Lateral digital extensor m.

5

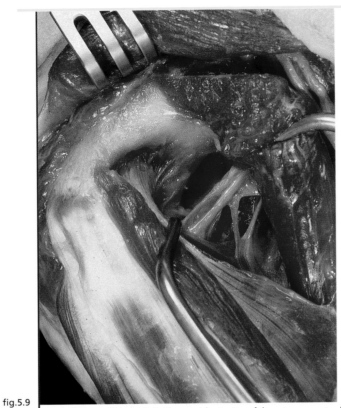

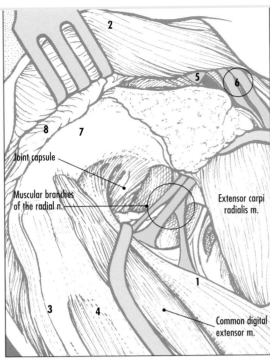

1 - Supinator m. **2** - Triceps brachii m. (lateral head) **3** - Extensor carpi ulnaris m. **4** - Lateral digital extensor m. **5** - Deep branch of the radial n. **6** - Superficial branches of the radial n. **7** - Lateral supracondylar crest. **8** - Anconeus m.

fig.5.9

Magnified view of figure 5.8. After cranial retraction of the extensor carpi radialis muscle, it is possible to identify the cranial aspect of the elbow joint and muscular branches of the radial nerve.

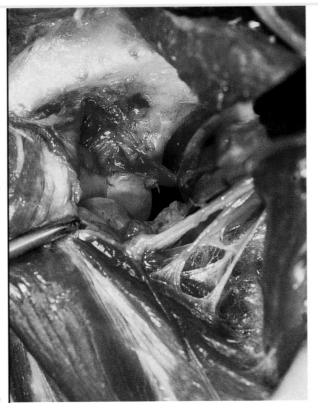

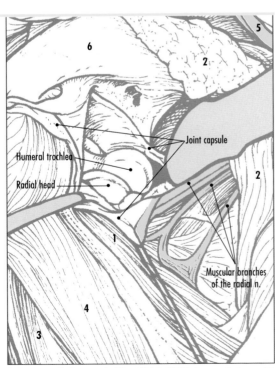

1 - Supinator m. **2** - Extensor carpi radialis m. **3** - Lateral digital extensor m. **4** - Common digital extensor m. **5** - Superficial branches of the radial n. **6** - Lateral supracondylar crest.

fig.5.10

Once the joint is opened, the anterior aspect of the humeral trochlea and radial head can be seen.

OSTEOTOMY OF THE LATERAL HUMERAL EPICONDYLE

5

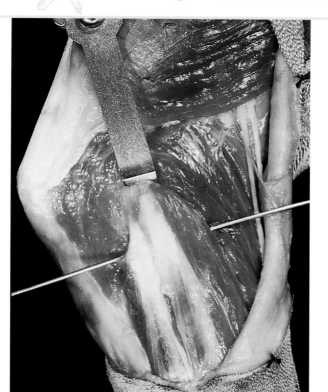

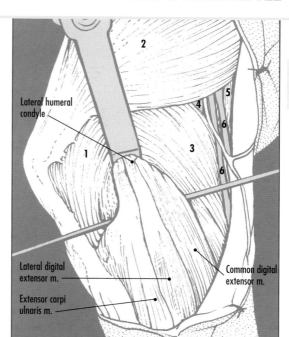

An intercondylar lag screw is used to reattach the epicondyle.

Lateral humeral condyle

Lateral digital extensor m.

Common digital extensor m.

Extensor carpi ulnaris m.

1 - Anconeus m. 2. Triceps brachii m. (lateral head) 3. Extensor carpi radialis m. 4. Deep branch of the radial n. 5. Brachialis m. 6. Superficial branches of the radial n.

fig.5.11

The initial steps of this approach are the same as described previously (see figs 5.1, 5.2, 5.3 and 5.4). Once the tendons of the extensor carpi ulnaris, lateral digital extensor and common digital extensor muscles have been identified, the lateral epicondyle is osteotomized, ensuring that the area of insertion of these muscles is attached to the separated epicondyle. The osteotomy plane is parallel to the radius.

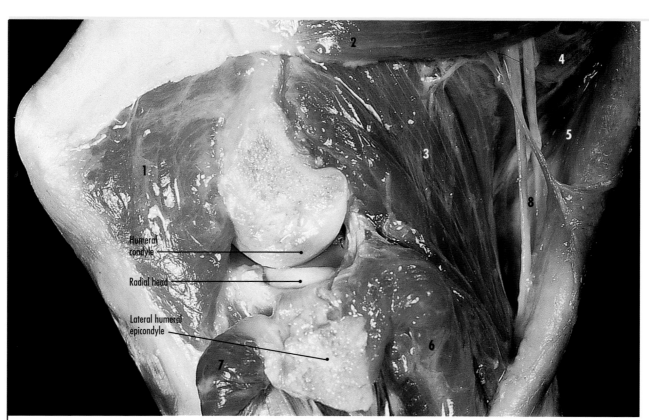

Humeral condyle

Radial head

Lateral humeral epicondyle

fig.5.12

The lateral aspect of the elbow joint is reached after the lateral epicondyle and its muscular insertion has been retracted distally and arthrotomy has been performed.

1 - Anconeus m. 2 - Triceps brachii m. (lateral head) 3 - Extensor carpi radialis m. 4 - Brachialis m. 5 - Cephalic v. 6 - Common digital extensor m. 7 - Extensor carpi ulnaris m. 8 - Superficial branches of the radial n.

5

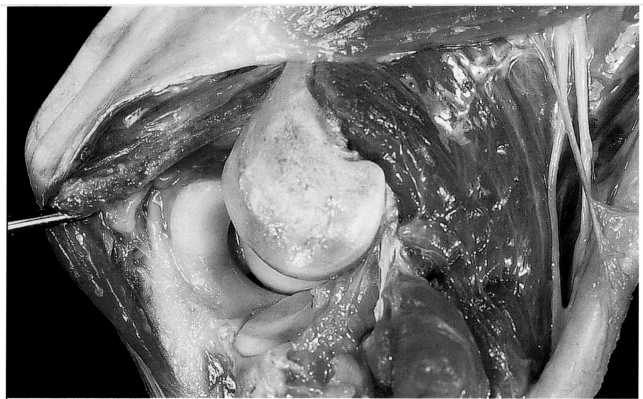

fig.5.13

External rotation and adduction of the antebrachium allows greater exposure of the articular surfaces of the humerus, ulna and radius.

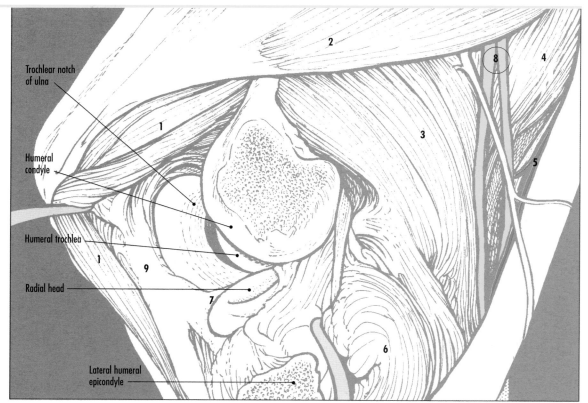

Trochlear notch of ulna

Humeral condyle

Humeral trochlea

Radial head

Lateral humeral epicondyle

1 - Anconeus m. **2** - Triceps brachii m. (lateral head) **3** - Extensor carpi radialis m. **4** - Brachialis m. **5** - Cephalic v. **6** - Common digital extensor m. **7** - Lateral coronoid process of the ulna **8** - Superficial branches of the radial n. **9** - Olecranon

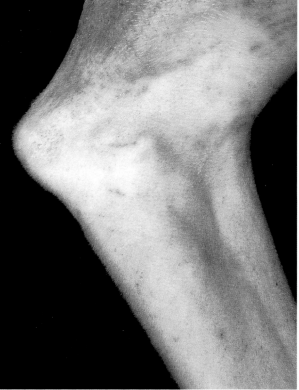

fig.6.1

The animal is in left lateral recumbency. Medial view of the left thoracic limb

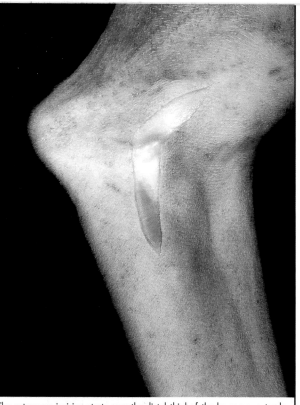

fig.6.2

The cutaneous incision starts over the distal third of the humerus, extends distally over the medial epicondyle and finishes at the proximal third of the radius.

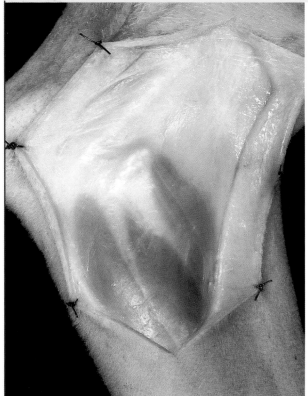

fig.6.3

Triceps brachii m.
(medial head)

1 - Pronator teres m. **2** - Flexor carpi radialis m. **3** - Superficial digital flexor m.

Subcutaneous tissue and superficial fascia are incised and retracted in the same fashion. The deep fascia is incised in the same way, avoiding the ulnar nerve located underneath it, following the cranial border of the medial head of the triceps brachii muscle.

INTERMUSCULAR

6

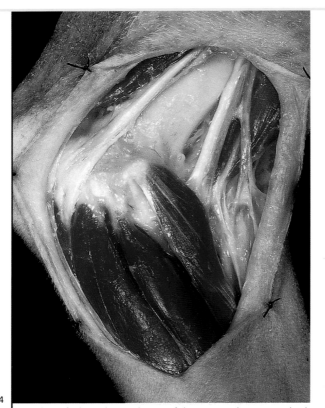

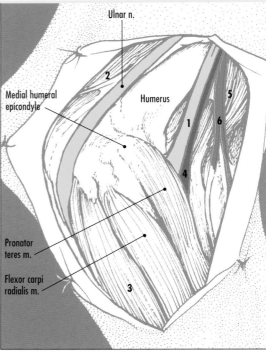

Ulnar n.

Medial humeral
epicondyle

Humerus

Pronator
teres m.

Flexor carpi
radialis m.

1 - Median n. 2 - Triceps brachii m. (medial head) 3 - Superficial digital flexor m. 4 - Brachial
a. 5 - Biceps brachii m. 6 - Superficial brachial a. and v.

fig.6.4

In order to facilitate the visualisation of the anatomical structures, the deep fascia has been removed. Fatty tissue has to be removed to gain access to the medial epicondylar area. The medial epicondyle, pronator teres muscle and flexor carpi radialis muscle have to be identified in the approach to the medial coronoid process.

Intermuscular dissection can be performed between the flexor carpi radialis muscle and the superficial and deep digital flexor muscles.

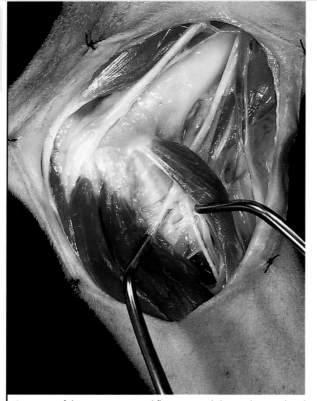

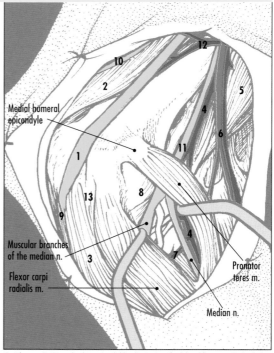

Medial humeral
epicondyle

Muscular branches
of the median n.

Flexor carpi
radialis m.

Pronator
teres m.

Median n.

1 - Ulnar n. 2 - Triceps brachii m. (medial head) 3 - Superficial digital flexor m. 4 - Brachial a.
5 - Biceps brachii m. 6 - Superficial brachial a. and v. 7 - Common interosseous a. 8 - Joint capsule 9 - Flexor carpi ulnaris m. 10 - Caudal cutaneous antebrachial n. 11 - Median n. 12 - Collateral ulnar a. 13 - Deep digital flexor m.

fig.6.5

Separation of the pronator teres and flexor carpi radialis muscles, avoiding damage to the median nerve and its muscular branches, allows visualisation of the joint capsule, covered by the tendinous insertion of the brachialis and biceps brachii muscles.

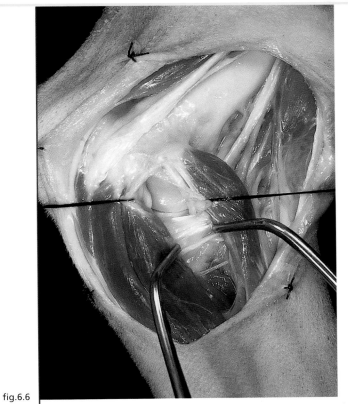

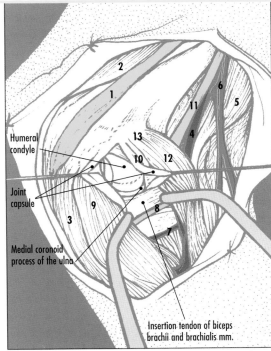

Humeral condyle

Joint capsule

Medial coronoid process of the ulna

Insertion tendon of biceps brachii and brachialis mm.

1 -Ulnar n. **2** -Triceps brachii m. (medial head) **3** -Superficial digital flexor m. **4** -Brachial a.
5 - Biceps brachii m. **6** -Superficial brachial a. and v. **7** -Common interosseous a. **8** -Muscular branch of the median n. **9** -Flexor carpi radialis m. **10** -Medial collateral ligament **11** -Median n.
12 -Pronator teres m. **13** -Medial humeral epicondyle

fig.6.6

The joint capsule is incised parallel to the flexor muscles, allowing access to the intra-articular structures.

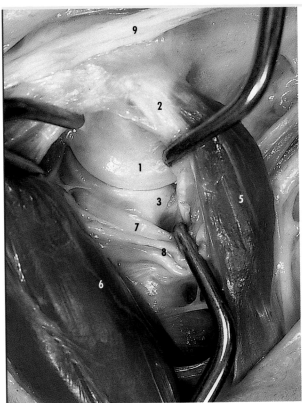

fig.6.7

Proper separation of the articular capsule, flexor muscles and the insertion tendon of the biceps brachii and brachialis muscles by a pair of Gelpi retractors allows examination of the area of the medial coronoid process. Outward and inward rotation of the limb improves the visualisation of the anatomical structures.

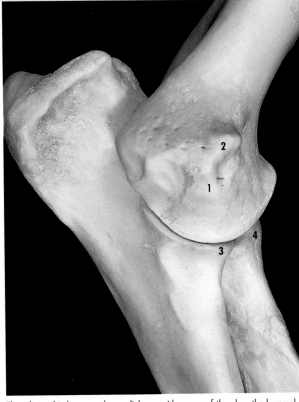

A sandbag under the lateral aspect of the elbow creates a fulcrum that helps the visualization of the articular aspect of the coronoid process.

Key to figs. 6.7 and 6.8

1 - Humeral condyle

2 - Medial humeral epicondyle

3 - Medial coronoid process of the ulna

4 - Radial head

5 - Pronator teres m.

6 - Flexor carpi radialis m.

7 - Insertion tendon of the biceps brachii and brachialis mm.

8 - Muscular branches of the median n.

9 - Ulnar n

fig.6.8

The relationship between the medial coronoid process of the ulna, the humeral condyle and the head of the radius can be observed above.

OSTEOTOMY OF THE MEDIAL HUMERAL EPICONDYLE

6

The separated epicondyle is fixed with a lag screw. Drilling and tapping the screw hole is carried out before the osteotomy is performed, facilitating the re-attachment of the epicondyle.

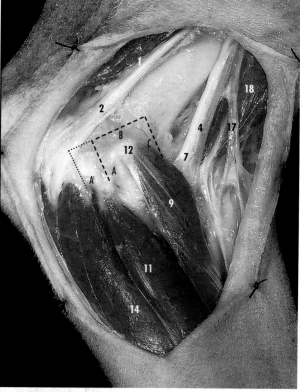

fig.6.9

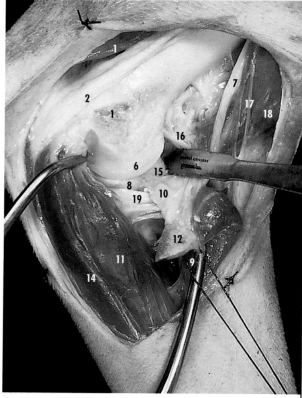

fig.6.10

The initial steps of this approach are the same as those described previously (see figures 6.1., 6.2 and 6.3). Osteotomy is performed by means of three incisions using a chisel and involves the area of origin of the pronator teres and flexor carpi radialis muscles[1]. The first cut (caudal to the epicondyle) (**A** or **A´**)[1] and the second cut (proximal) (**B**) are about 5mm deep and perpendicular to the bone; the third cut (cranial) (**C**) involves the use of the chisel in a horizontal fashion, until it connects the other two and frees the bony fragment (see key on page 33).

[1] In larger breeds of dog, the pronator teres and flexor carpi radialis muscles are relatively distant from each other and as a consequence of this, a larger area would be separated. Sufficient access to the joint may be obtained by separating only that part of the epicondyle where the pronator teres muscle has its origin. This fragment is large enough to accommodate the lag screw, when closure is performed.

The joint is visualised after distal reflection of the separated epicondyle, pronator teres and flexor carpi radialis muscles, and the medial collateral ligament, followed by incision of the articular capsule. In this photo, the tendon of the flexor carpi radialis muscle has not been involved in the osteotomy (see key on page 33).

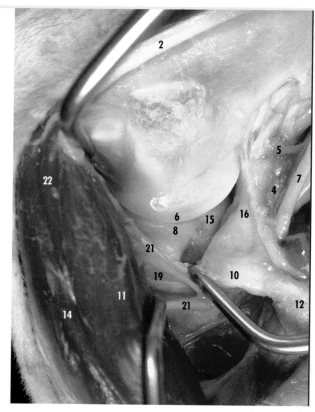

Visualisation of the medial coronoid process is improved by ventral reflection of the insertion of the biceps brachii and brachialis muscles as well as pronation and supination of the limb (see key on page 33).

fig.6.11

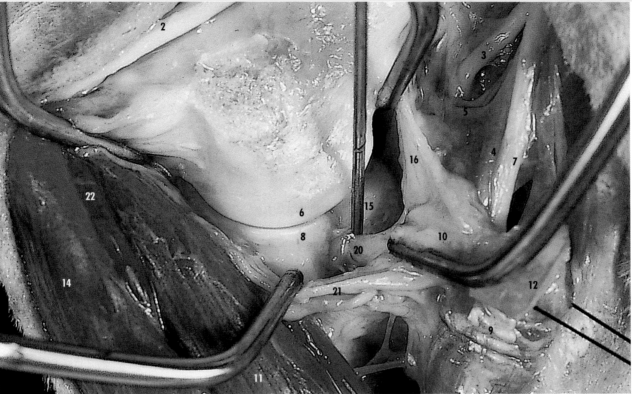

fig.6.12

Magnified view of the area showing the annular ligament of the radius, deep to the medial coronoid process.

THORACIC LIMB

Key to figs. 6.9 to 6.13

1 - Triceps brachii m. (medial head)	**13** - Antebrachial fascia
	14 - Superficial digital flexor m.
2 - Ulnar n.	**15** - Radial head
3 - Musculocutaneous n.	**16** - Articular capsule
4 - Brachial a.	**17** - Superficial brachial a. and v.
5 - Transverse cubital a.	
6 - Humeral trochlea	**18** - Biceps brachii m.
7 - Median n.	**19** - Insertion tendon of the biceps brachii and brachialis mm.
8 - Medial coronoid process	
9 - Pronator teres m.	**20** - Radial annular ligament
10 - Medial collateral ligament	**21** - Muscular branches of the median n.
11 - Flexor carpi radialis m.	**22** - Deep digital flexor m.
12 - Medial humeral epicondyle	

fig.6.13

The use of a sandbag placed under the lateral aspect of the elbow creates a fulcrum that helps the visualisation of the articular surfaces. In this picture, the origin of the tendon of the flexor carpi radialis muscle is also included with the separated epicondyle.

33

MEDIAL APPROACH TO THE FELINE ELBOW

■ The medial epicondylar region of the cat has some anatomical features that warrant the following approach.

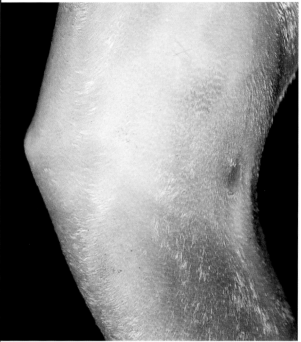

fig.6.14

The animal is in left lateral recumbency. Medial view of the left thoracic limb.

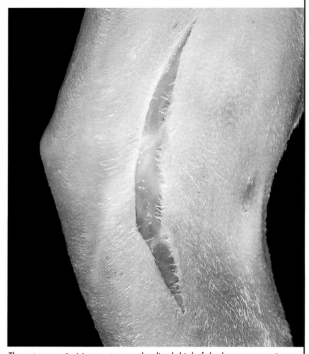

fig.6.15

The cutaneous incision starts over the distal third of the humerus, continues above the medial epicondyle and finishes at the proximal third of the radius.

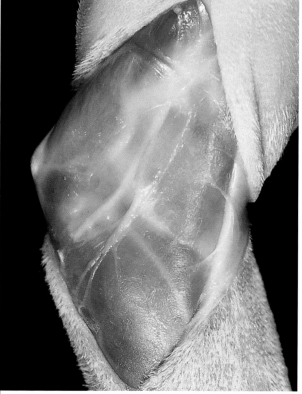

fig.6.16

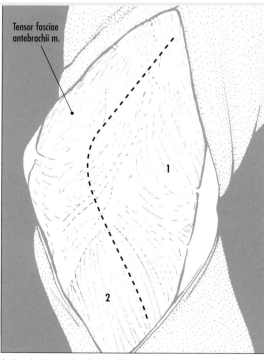

Tensor fasciae antebrachii m.

1 - Biceps brachii m. 2 - Superficial digital flexor m.

Subcutaneous tissue and superficial fascia are incised and retracted in the same fashion. The deep fascia is incised in the same way, avoiding the ulnar nerve located underneath it.

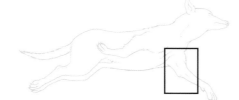

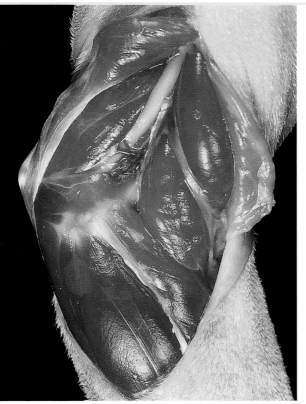

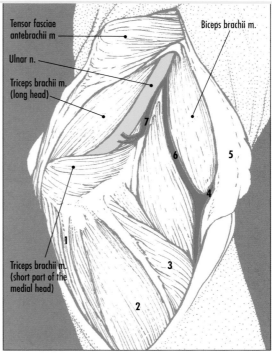

1 - Flexor carpi ulnaris m. 2 - Superficial digital flexor m. 3 - Pronator teres m. 4 - Median cubital v. 5 - Brachiocephalicus m. 6 - Brachial v. 7 - Collateral ulnar v.

fig.6.17

The biceps brachii and triceps brachii muscles are exposed after incising the deep fascia and caudally retracting the tensor fasciae antebrachii muscle. The triceps brachii muscle is then retracted caudally and the biceps brachii muscle is retracted cranially. The ulnar nerve is retracted with the triceps brachii muscle.

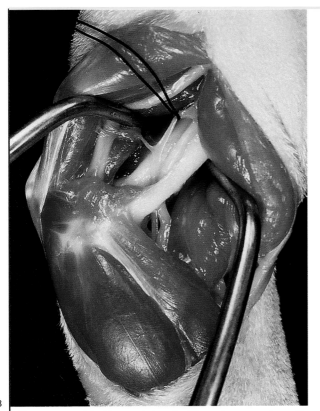

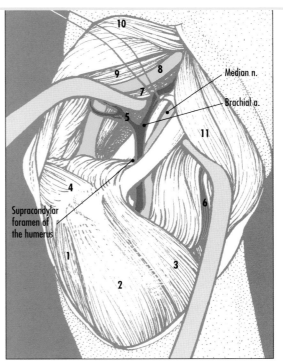

1 - Flexor carpi ulnaris m. 2 - Superficial digital flexor m. 3 - Pronator teres m. 4 - Triceps brachii m. (short part of the medial head) 5 - Collateral ulnar a. 6 - Brachial v. 7 - Triceps brachii m. (medial head) 8 - Ulnar n. 9 - Triceps brachii m. (long head) 10 - Tensor fasciae antebrachii m. 11 - Biceps brachii m.

fig.6.18

The separation of the biceps and triceps brachii muscles exposes the median nerve and brachial artery that cross the supracondylar foramen of the elbow humerus.

THORACIC LIMB

APPENDIX

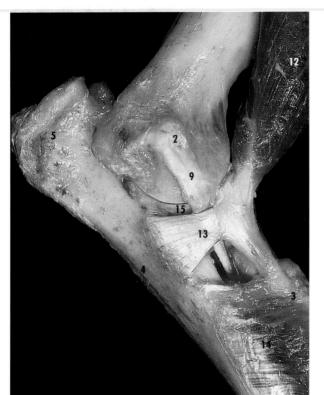

fig.6.19

Anatomical dissection of the medial aspect of the elbow joint. Observe the close relationship between the medial collateral ligament and the tendon of insertion of the brachialis and biceps brachii muscles, which lie over the medial coronoid process.

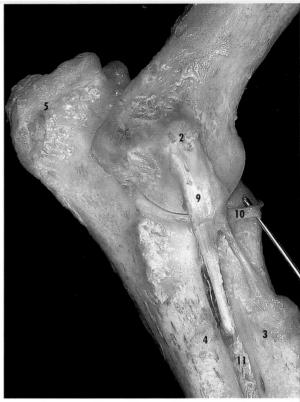

fig.6.20

Anatomical dissection of the medial aspect of the elbow joint. The tendon of insertion of the brachialis and biceps brachii muscles has been removed, showing the medial collateral ligament and the annular ligament of the radius.

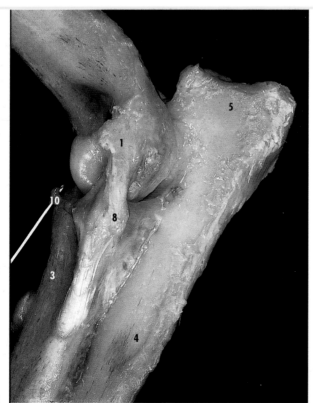

fig.6.21

Anatomical dissection of the lateral aspect of the elbow, showing the lateral collateral ligament and the annular ligament of the radius.

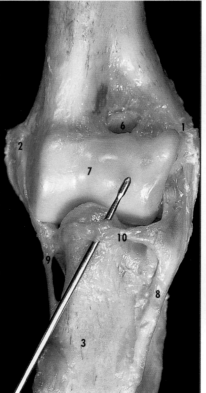

fig.6.22

Anatomical dissection of the cranial aspect of the elbow, showing the annular ligament of the radius and the collateral ligaments of the joint.

Key to figs. 6.19 to 6.22

1 - Lateral humeral epicondyle
2 - Medial humeral epicondyle
3 - Radius
4 - Ulna
5 - Olecranon tuberosity
6 - Supratrochlear foramen
7 - Trochlea of the humerus
8 - Lateral collateral ligament
9 - Medial collateral ligament
10 - Annular ligament of the radius
11 - Interosseous membrane of the antebrachium
12 - Biceps brachii m.
13 - Insertion tendon of brachialis and biceps brachii mm.
14 - Pronator quadratus m.
15 - Medial coronoid process

Approach to the Elbow Joint by Osteotomy of the Tuber Olecrani[1]

7

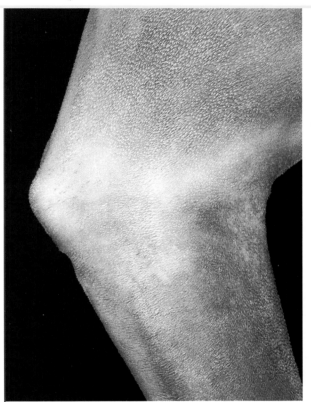

fig.7.1

The animal is in partial left lateral recumbency, allowing access to both lateral and medial aspects of the elbow. Lateral view of the right elbow.

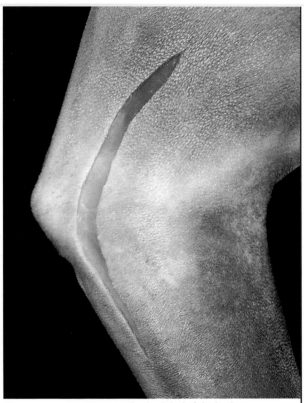

fig.7.2

The cutaneous incision starts in the distal third of the brachium, continues caudally over the lateral humeral epicondyle and finishes in the middle third of the antebrachium.

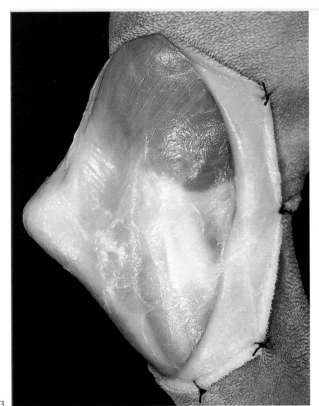

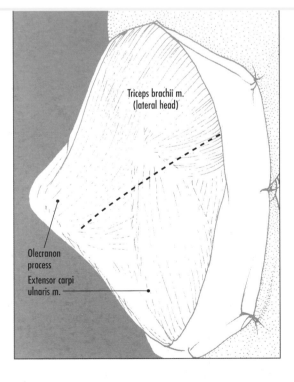

Triceps brachii m.
(lateral head)

Olecranon process

Extensor carpi ulnaris m.

fig.7.3

Subcutaneous tissue and superficial fascia are incised and retracted on both the lateral and medial aspects of the elbow, exposing both sides of the olecranon. The deep fascia is incised following the cranial edge of the lateral head of the triceps brachii muscle.

[1] Also known as the olecranon.

7

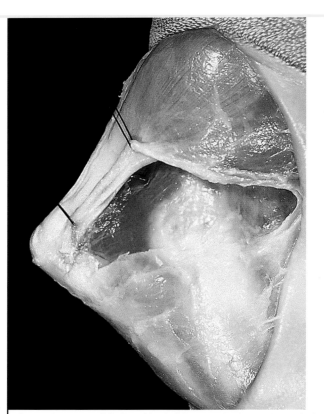

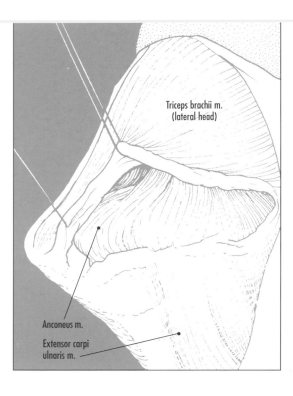

Triceps brachii m.
(lateral head)

Anconeus m.

Extensor carpi
ulnaris m.

fig.7.4

The dorsal retraction of the lateral head of the triceps brachii muscle reveals the anconeus muscle, which will be separated from the proximal ulna.

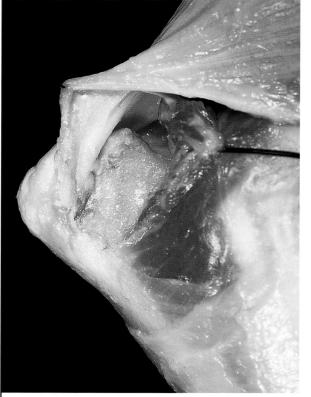

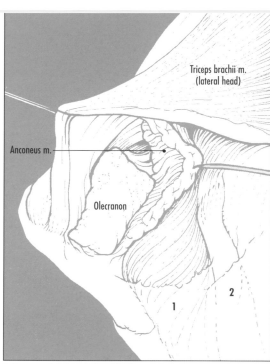

Triceps brachii m.
(lateral head)

Anconeus m.

Olecranon

1   2

1 - Extensor carpi ulnaris m.   2 - Lateral digital extensor m.

fig.7.5

Once the anconeus muscle has been reflected cranially, the lateral aspect of the olecranon and the tendon of insertion of the triceps brachii muscle are identified.

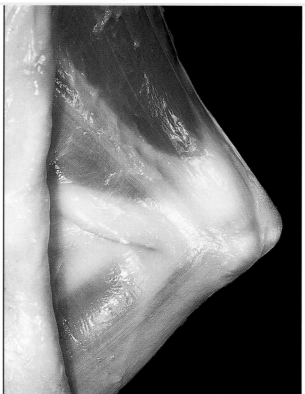

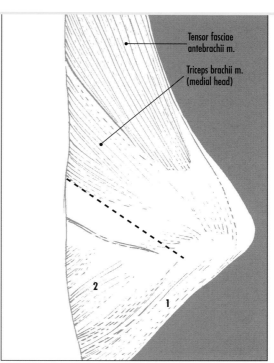

1 - Flexor carpi ulnaris m. (ulnar head) 2 - Superficial digital flexor m.

fig.7.6

Medial view of the right elbow. The approach is continued on the medial aspect by identifying the tensor fasciae antebrachii muscle and the lateral and long heads of the triceps brachii muscle. An incision in the fascia will be made, following the cranial border of the medial head. The ulnar nerve is palpable through the fascia, avoiding injury.

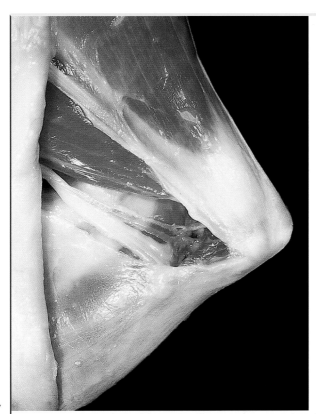

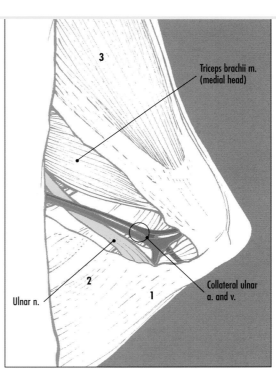

1 - Flexor carpi ulnaris m. (ulnar head) 2 - Superficial digital flexor m. 3 - Tensor fasciae antebrachii m.

fig.7.7

The ulnar nerve is identified and dissected to allow its retraction away from the osteotomy site.

7

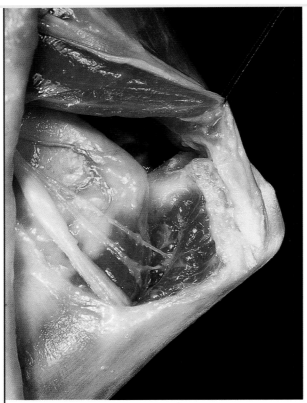

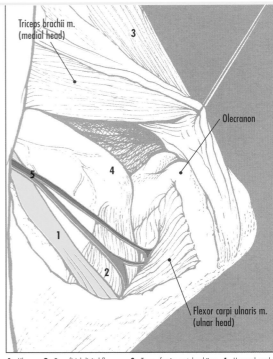

Triceps brachii m.
(medial head)

3

Olecranon

5

4

1

2

Flexor carpi ulnaris m.
(ulnar head)

1 - Ulnar n. **2** - Superficial digital flexor m. **3** - Tensor fasciae antebrachii m. **4** - Humeral condyle **5** - Collateral ulnar a. and v.

fig.7.8

Proximal retraction of the belly of the triceps brachii muscle isolates the insertion of its tendon and exposes the medial aspect of the olecranon, partially covered by the flexor carpi ulnaris muscle (ulnar head). Afterwards, this muscle will be incised to position the Gigli wire.

Key to
figs. 7.9 and 7.10

1 - Triceps brachii m.
(lateral head)

2 - Olecranon

3 - Anconeus m.

4 - Anconeal process of
the ulna

5 - Lateral coronoid
process of the ulna

6 - Lateral humeral
epicondyle

7 - Radial head

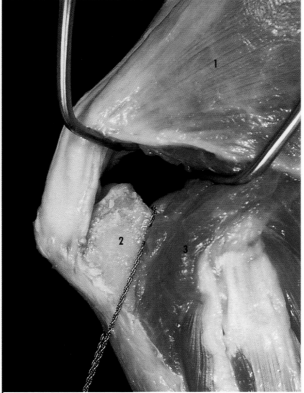

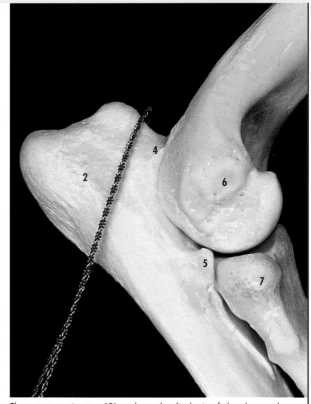

fig.7.9

Lateral view of the right elbow, showing the Gigli wire being passed under the triceps brachii tendon and against the base of the anconeal process of the ulna.

fig.7.10

The osteotomy is at a 45° angle to the diaphysis of the ulna as shown above.

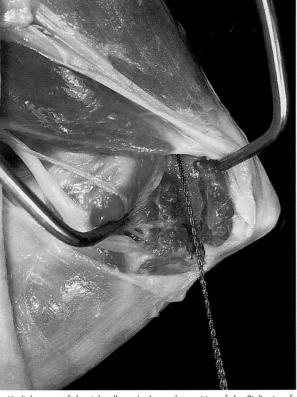

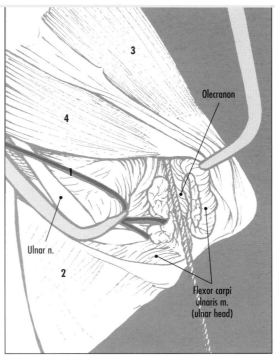

1 - Collateral ulnar vessels **2** - Superficial digital flexor m. **3** - Tensor fasciae antebrachii m.
4 - Triceps brachii m. (medial head)

fig.7.11

Medial aspect of the right elbow. It shows the position of the Gigli wire after the flexor carpi ulnaris muscle (ulnar head) has been incised. It is very important to ensure the ulnar nerve has been kept away from the site of the osteotomy.

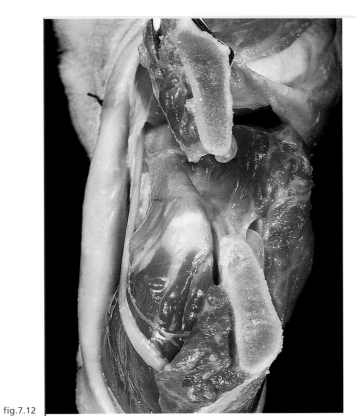

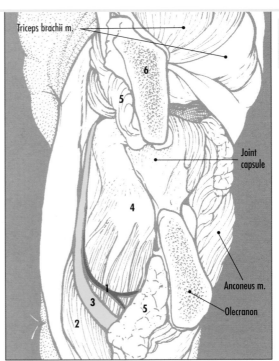

The osteotomized fragment is reattached with a tensión band device.

1 - Collateral ulnar vessels. 2. Superficial digital flexor m. 3. Ulnar n. 4. Humeral condyle 5. Flexor carpi ulnaris m. (ulnar head) 6. Olecranon

fig.7.12

Dorsal view of the right elbow after osteotomy. The olecranon fossa (together with the anconeus muscle), and the joint capsule are exposed after the proximal retraction of the olecranon and triceps brachii muscle.

7

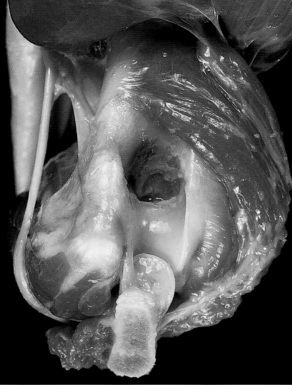

fig.7.13

Arthrotomy allows access to the caudal aspect of the elbow joint.

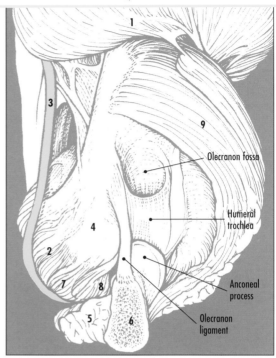

Olecranon fossa

Humeral trochlea

Anconeal process

Olecranon ligament

1 - Triceps brachii m. **2** - Superficial digital flexor m. **3** - Ulnar n. **4** - Humeral condyle **5** - Flexor carpi ulnaris m. (ulnar head) **6** - Olecranon **7** - Flexor carpi ulnaris m. (humeral head) **8** - Deep digital flexor m. (humeral head) **9** - Anconeus m. **10** - Humeral trochlea **11** - Olecranon ligament **12** - Supratrochlear foramen.

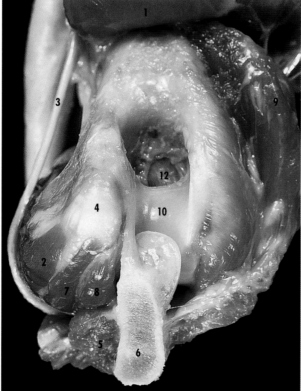

fig.7.14

The exposure of the supracondylar region improves with retraction of the anconeus muscle (see key to fig 7.13).

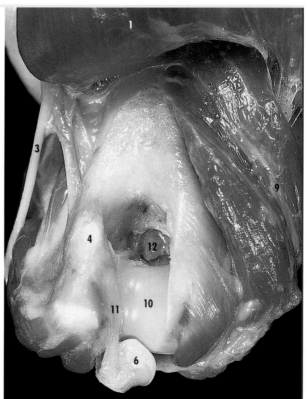

fig.7.15

Elbow hyperflexion improves the visualisation of the humeral trochlea (see key to fig 7.13).

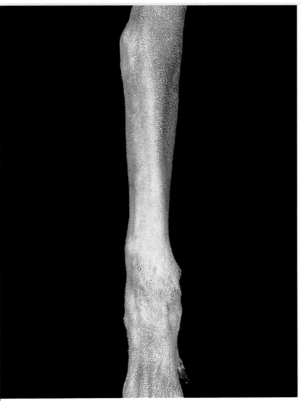

fig.8.1

The animal is in sternal recumbency. Dorsal view of the right thoracic limb.

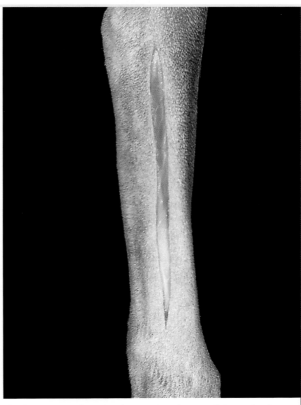

Compression of the proximal aspect of the cranial antebrachium helps to raise the cephalic vein, thereby improving its visualisation during the skin incision.

fig.8.2

The skin incision is located in the craniolateral aspect of the antebrachium.

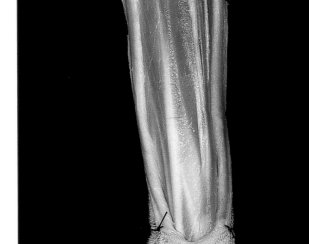

fig.8.3

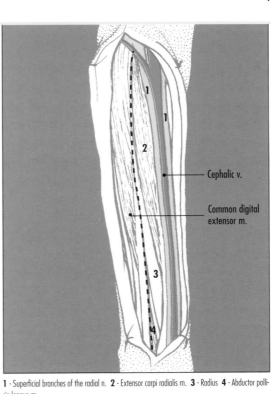

Cephalic v.

Common digital extensor m.

1 - Superficial branches of the radial n. **2** - Extensor carpi radialis m. **3** - Radius **4** - Abductor pollicis longus m.

The subcutaneous tissue and superficial fascia are incised in the same fashion. The deep fascia is incised, following the cranial margin of the common digital extensor muscle.

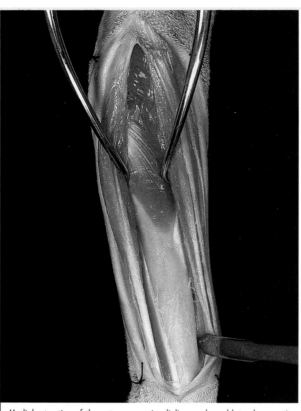

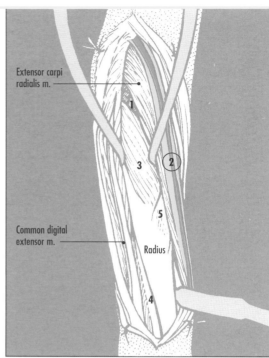

1 - Deep branch of the radial n. 2 - Superficial branches of the radial n., cephalic v. 3 - Supinator m. 4 - Abductor pollicis longus m. 5 - Insertion of the pronator teres m.

fig.8.4

Medial retraction of the extensor carpi radialis muscle and lateral separation of the common digital extensor and lateral digital extensor muscles allows exposure of most of the cranial aspect of the shaft of the radius.

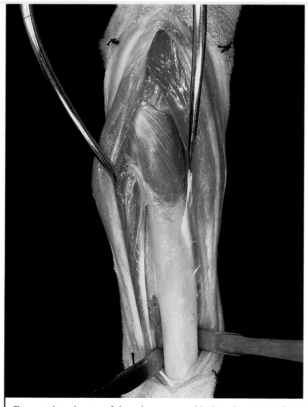

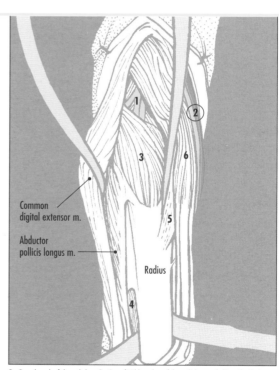

1 - Deep branch of the radial n. 2 - Superficial branches of the radial n., cephalic v. 3 - Supinator m. 4 - Interosseous space. 5 - Insertion of the pronator teres m. 6 - Extensor carpi radialis m.

fig.8.5

The craniolateral region of the radius is exposed by lateral retraction of the abductor pollicis longus m.

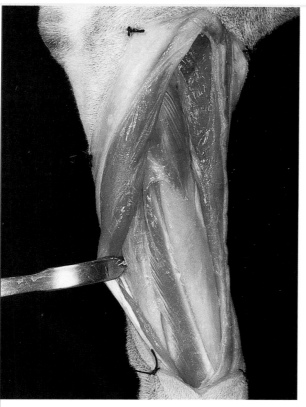

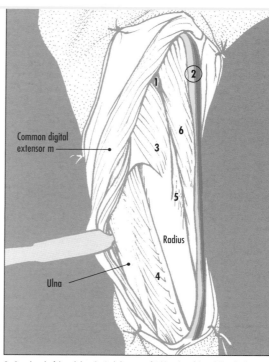

Common digital
extensor m

Radius

Ulna

1 - Deep branch of the radial n. 2 - Cephalic v., superficial branches of the radial n. 3 - Supinator
m. 4 - Abductor pollicis longus m. 5 - Insertion of the pronator teres m. 6 - Extensor carpi radialis m.

fig.8.6

The approach to the ulnar shaft requires caudolateral retraction of the common digital extensor muscle.

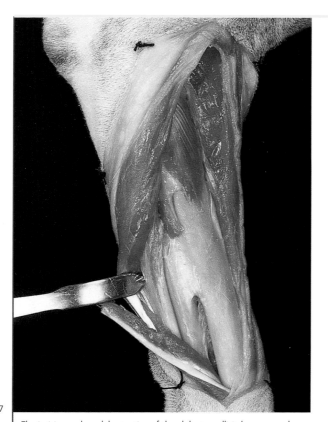

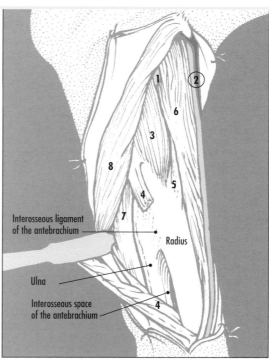

The approach to the
radius can be increased
proximally by partial or
complete incision of the
insertion of the supinator
muscle. This will be sutured
with the pronator teres
muscle at closure.

Interosseous ligament
of the antebrachium

Radius

Ulna

Interosseous space
of the antebrachium

1 - Deep branch of the radial n. 2 - Cephalic v., superficial branches of the radial n. 3 - Supinator
m. 4 - Abductor pollicis longus m. 5 - Insertion of the pronator teres m. 6 - Extensor carpi radialis m. 7 - Lateral digital extensor m. 8 - Common digital extensor m.

fig.8.7

The incision and caudal retraction of the abductor pollicis longus muscle exposes the interosseous ligament and space of the antebrachium.

Dorsal Approach
to the Distal Radius and Carpus

9

Compression of the proximal aspect of the cranial antebrachium helps to raise the cephalic and accessory cephalic veins, improving visualisation during the skin incision.

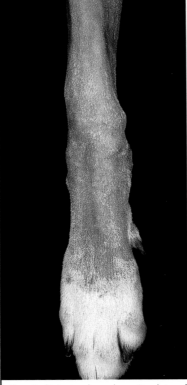

fig.9.1

The animal is in sternal recumbency. Dorsal view of the right thoracic limb.

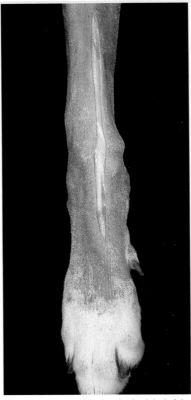

The cutaneous incision starts at the distal third of the cranial aspect of the antebrachium and extends to the middle third of metacarpal bone III.

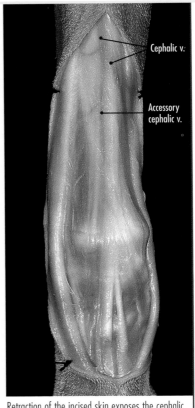

figs.9.2 and 9.3

Cephalic v.

Accessory cephalic v.

Retraction of the incised skin exposes the cephalic and accessory cephalic veins. Incision of the superficial fascia parallel to the veins allows them to be separated.

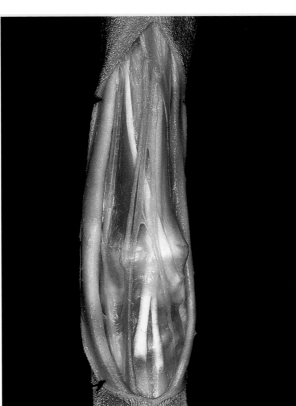

fig.9.4

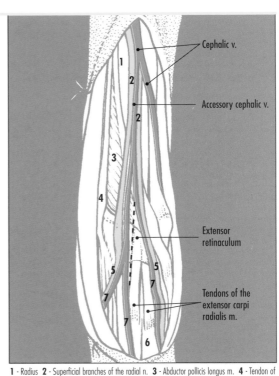

Cephalic v.

Accessory cephalic v.

Extensor retinaculum

Tendons of the extensor carpi radialis m.

1 - Radius **2** - Superficial branches of the radial n. **3** - Abductor pollicis longus m. **4** - Tendon of the common digital extensor m. **5** - Dorsal common digital nn. **6** - Metacarpal bone II **7** - Dorsal common digital vv.

The image shows the area of interest after most of the deep fascia has been removed in order to improve visualisation of the anatomical structures. The extensor retinaculum will be incised lateral to the tendons of the extensor carpi radialis muscle.

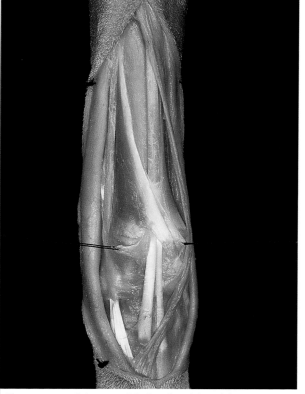

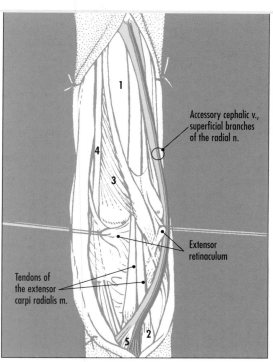

The cranial superficial antebrachial artery accompanies the cephalic and accessory cephalic veins, but due to its small size, is difficult to visualize.

Accessory cephalic v., superficial branches of the radial n.

Extensor retinaculum

Tendons of the extensor carpi radialis m.

1 - Radius 2 - Metacarpal bone II 3 - Abductor pollicis longus m. 4 - Tendon of the common digital extensor m. 5 - Metacarpal bone III

fig.9.5

The accessory cephalic vein and the branches of the radial nerve are retracted medially. The extensor retinaculum is opened, allowing visualisation of the tendons of the extensor carpi radialis muscle.

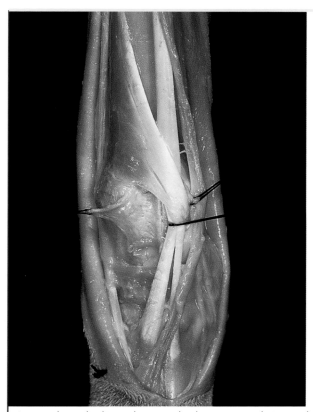

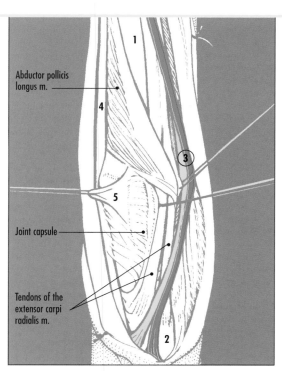

Abductor pollicis longus m.

Joint capsule

Tendons of the extensor carpi radialis m.

1 - Radius 2 - Metacarpal II 3 - Accessory cephalic v. and superficial branches of the radial n.
4 - Tendon of the common digital extensor m. 5 - Extensor retinaculum

fig.9.6

Access to the antebrachiocarpal, intercarpal and carpometacarpal joints is achieved by retraction of the extensor carpi radialis and abductor pollicis longus muscles.

9

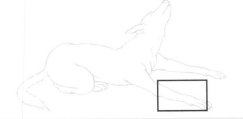

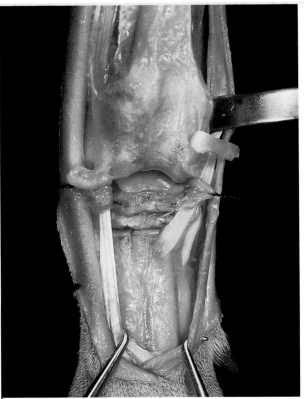

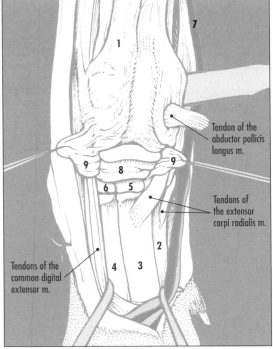

1 - Radius 2 - Metacarpal II 3 - Metacarpal III 4 - Metacarpal IV 5 - Carpal bone III 6 - Carpal bone IV 7 - Accessory cephalic v. and superficial branches of the radial n. 8 - Radial carpal bone (scaphoid) 9 - Joint capsule

Tendon of the abductor pollicis longus m.

Tendons of the extensor carpi radialis m.

Tendons of the common digital extensor m.

fig.9.7

Application of a bone plate for pancarpal arthrodesis requires incision of the tendon of the abductor pollicis longus muscle, lateral retraction of the common digital extensor muscle and medial retraction of the extensor carpi radialis muscle. The picture shows some of the articular surfaces of the bones after incision of the articular capsule.

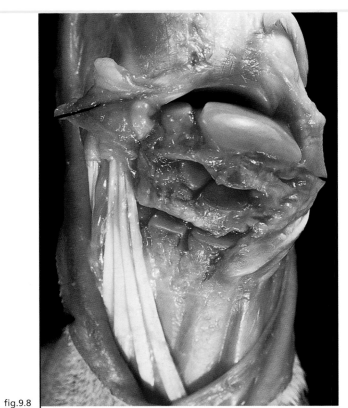

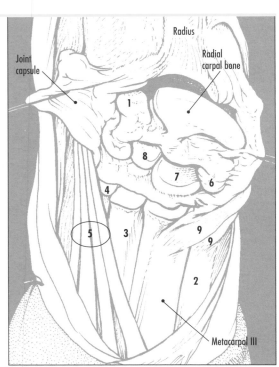

Radius

Joint capsule

Radial carpal bone

Metacarpal III

1 - Ulnar carpal bone 2 - Metacarpal II 3 - Metacarpal IV 4 - Metacarpal V 5 - Tendons of the common digital extensor m. 6 - Carpal bone II 7 - Carpal bone III 8 - Carpal bone IV 9 - Tendons of the extensor carpi radialis m

fig.9.8

The exposure of the different carpal bones, especially the radial carpal bone, and metacarpal bones, is achieved by carpal hyperflexion after incising the articular capsules and intercarpal and carpometacarpal ligaments.

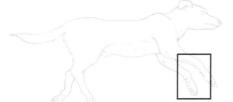

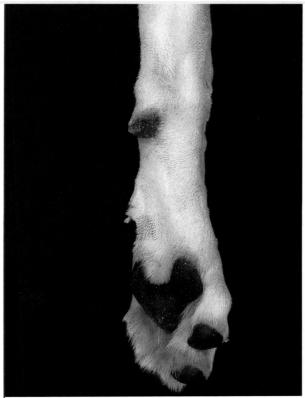

fig.10.1

The animal is in left lateral recumbency. Lateropalmar view of the right thoracic limb.

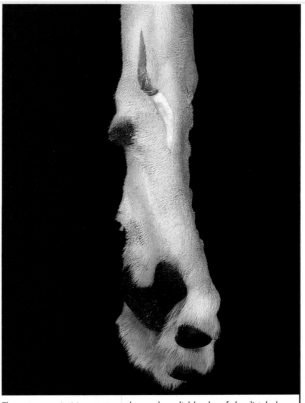

fig.10.2

The cutaneous incision starts at the caudomedial border of the distal ulna, follows the accessory carpal bone and the carpal pad, and finishes at the palmar aspect of the proximal third of metacarpal V.

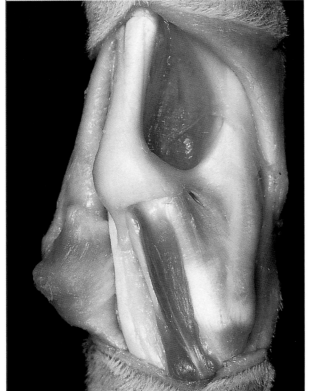

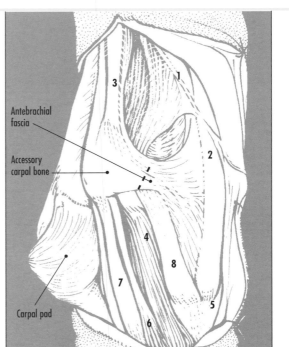

Antebrachial fascia

Accessory carpal bone

Carpal pad

1 - Dorsal branch of the ulnar n. **2** - Tendon of the extensor carpi ulnaris m. **3** - Tendon of the flexor carpi ulnaris m. **4** - Abductor digiti quinti m. **5** - Metacarpal V **6** - Flexor digiti quinti m. **7** - Tendon of the superficial digital flexor m. **8** - Accessory metacarpal ligament

fig.10.3

The subcutaneous tissue and superficial fascia are incised and retracted with the skin. To retract the carpal pad medially, an incision is made in the deep fascia where it joins the accessory carpal bone. Afterwards, the thickened fascia between the accessory carpal bone and the tendon of the extensor carpi ulnaris muscle will be incised.

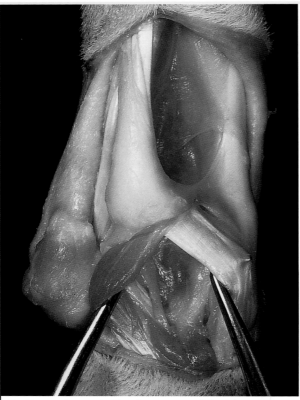

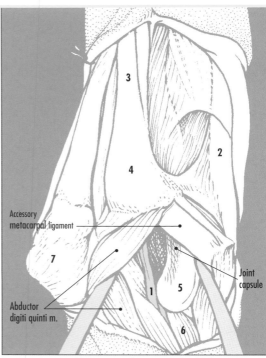

1 - Ulnar n. 2 - Tendon of the extensor carpi ulnaris m. 3 - Tendon of the flexor carpi ulnaris m.
4 - Accessory carpal bone 5 - Ulnar carpal bone 6 - Interosseous m. of digit V 7 - Carpal pad.

fig.10.4

The joint capsule is reached by palmar retraction of the abductor digiti quinti tendon and dorsal retraction of the accessory metacarpal ligament. The joint capsule is located among the accessory and ulnar carpal bones and the ulna.

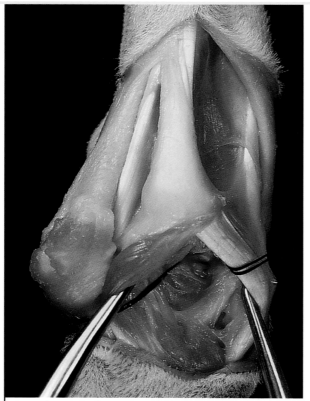

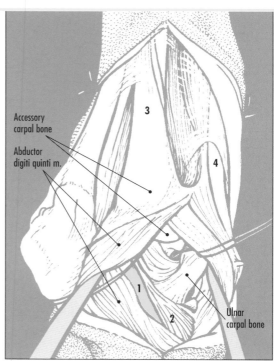

1 - Ulnar n. 2 - Interosseous m. of digit V 3 - Tendon of the flexor carpi ulnaris m. 4 - Tendon of the extensor carpi ulnaris m.

fig.10.5

Once arthrotomy has been performed, the articular surface of the accessory carpal bone is visualised. Access to the palmodistal aspect of the bone is improved by incising and retracting the abductor digiti quinti muscle.

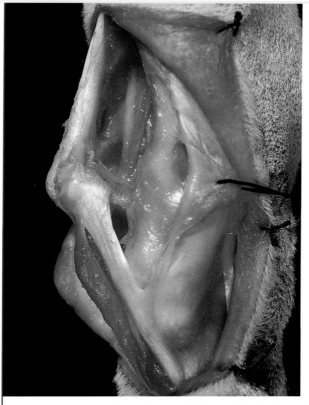

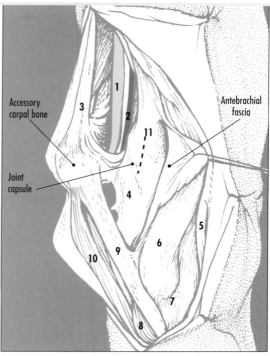

Accessory
carpal bone

Antebrachial
fascia

Joint
capsule

1 - Ulnar n. **2** - Caudal interosseous a. **3** - Tendon of the flexor carpi ulnaris m. **4** - Ulnar carpal bone **5** - Tendon of the lateral digital extensor m. **6** - Tendon of the extensor carpi ulnaris m. **7** - Metacarpal V **8** - Interosseous m. **9** - Accessory metacarpal ligament **10** - Abductor digiti quinti m. **11** - Lateral styloid process (ulna)

fig.10.6

Lateral view. The thickened band of antebrachial fascia is incised and retracted in order to gain access to the proximal border of the accessory carpal bone. Then, the joint capsule is identified and incised.

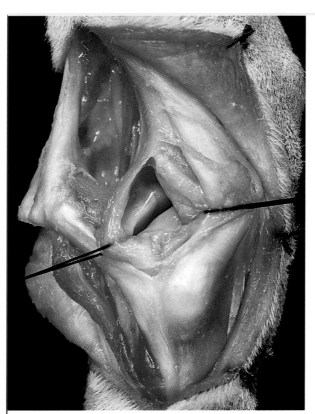

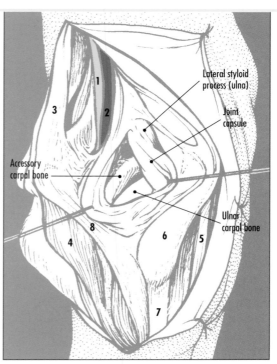

Lateral styloid
process (ulna)

Joint
capsule

Accessory
carpal bone

Ulnar
carpal bone

1 - Ulnar n. **2** - Caudal interosseous a. **3** - Tendon of the flexor carpi ulnaris m. **4** - Abductor digiti quinti m. **5** - Tendon of the lateral digital extensor m. **6** - Tendon of the extensor carpi ulnaris m. **7** - Metacarpal V **8** - Accessory metacarpal ligament.

fig.10.7

The retraction of the articular capsule allows visualization of the accessory carpal bone, ulnar carpal bone and ulna.

Dorsal Approach
to the Metacarpal Bones

11

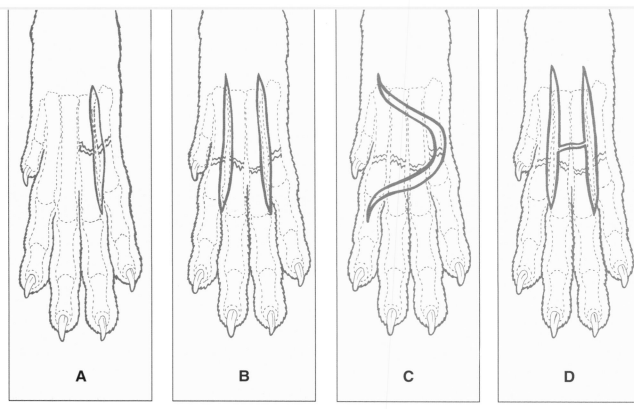

A

B

C

D

The cutaneous incision will depend on which metacarpal bone is approached. If only one metacarpal bone is involved, the incision will be made directly over it. If two are involved, the incision will be between them (A). If the four metacarpal bones are affected, different incisions are available (B, C, D) and also the incision performed as described below.

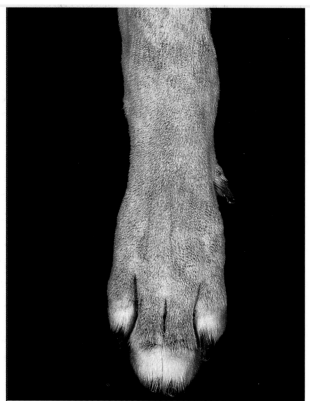

fig.11.1

The animal is in sternal recumbency. Dorsal view of the right thoracic paw

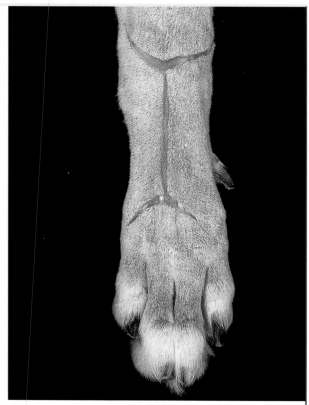

fig.11.2

The cutaneous incision to approach the four metacarpal bones is a laterally rotated "H".

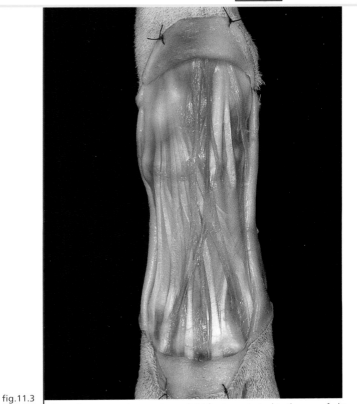

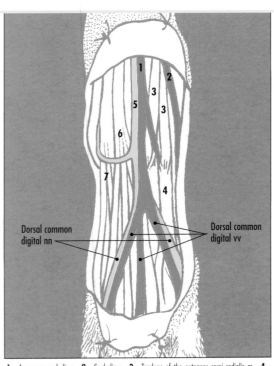

The dorsal common digital arteries accompany the veins and nerves of the same name, but due to their small size are difficult to identify.

Dorsal common digital nn.

Dorsal common digital vv.

1 - Accessory cephalic v. **2** - Cephalic v. **3** - Tendons of the extensor carpi radialis m. **4** - Metacarpal II **5** - Superficial branch of the radial n. **6** - Tendons of the common digital extensor m. **7** - Tendons of the lateral digital extensor m.

fig.11.3

The subcutaneous tissue and superficial fascia are incised in the same fashion, allowing visualisation of deeper structures, especially dorsal common digital veins and nerves. At this stage, small vascular and nervous structures may be incised without clinical significance.

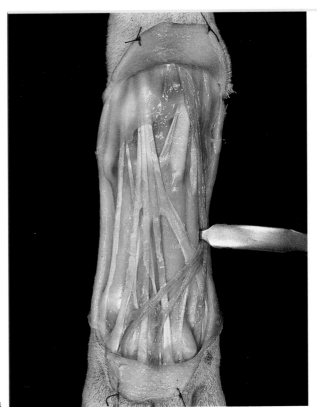

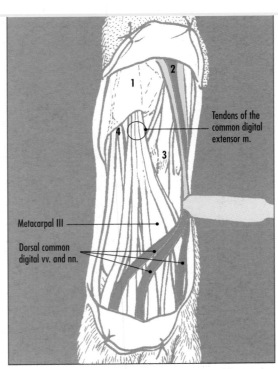

Tendons of the common digital extensor m.

Metacarpal III

Dorsal common digital vv. and nn.

1 - Extensor retinaculum **2** - Accessory cephalic v., superficial branches of the radial n. **3** - Tendons of the extensor carpi radialis m. **4** - Tendons of the lateral digital extensor m.

fig.11.4

The dorsal common digital veins and nerves are retracted medially, and then the tendons of the common digital extensor muscle are identified. The deep fascia has been removed to facilitate the view of the anatomical structures.

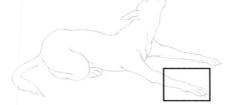

11

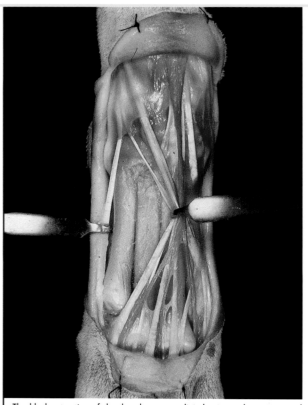

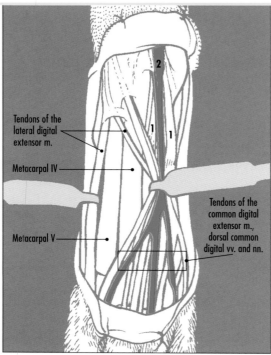

1 - Tendons of the extensor carpi radialis m. 2 - Accessory cephalic v., superficial branches of the radial n.

fig.11.5

The block retraction of the dorsal common digital veins and nerves, together with the common digital extensor muscle medially, and the tendons of the lateral digital extensor muscle laterally, allows access to metacarpal bones IV and V.

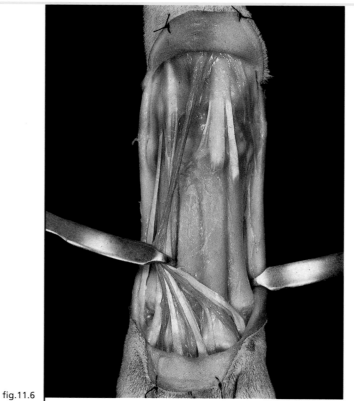

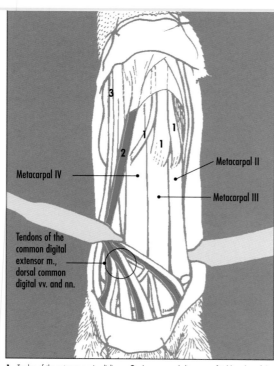

1 - Tendon of the extensor carpi radialis m. 2 - Accessory cephalic v., superficial branches of the radial n. 3 - Tendon of the lateral digital extensor m.

fig.11.6

The retraction of the dorsal common digital veins and nerves, together with the tendons of the common digital extensor muscle laterally, reveals the metacarpal bones II, III,IV.

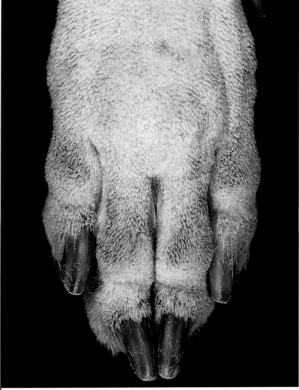

fig.12.1

The animal is in sternal recumbency. Dorsal view of the right thoracic paw.

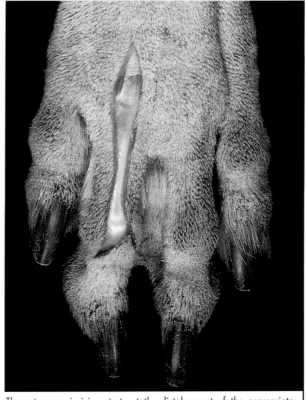

fig.12.2

The cutaneous incision starts at the distal aspect of the appropriate metacarpal bone (in this case, metacarpal IV) and extends distally to the medial or distal phalanges.

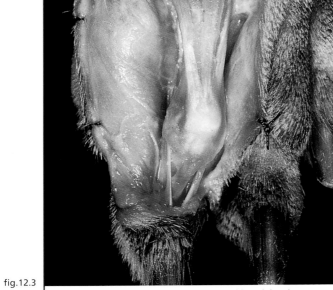

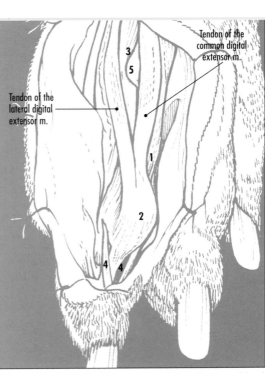

1 - Tendon of the interosseous m. of digit IV. 2 - Proximal interphalangeal joint 3 - Metacarpophalangeal joint 4 - Dorsal ligaments 5 - Dorsal sesamoid bone

fig.12.3

The tendons of the common digital extensor and lateral digital extensor muscles are seen overlying the proximal phalanx. During the approach, small neurovascular structures might be damaged, without any clinical implications.

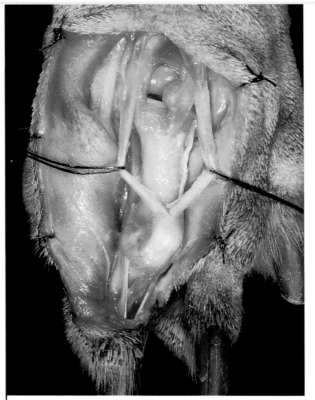

fig.12.4

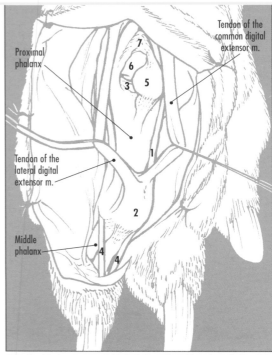

Tendon of the common digital extensor m.

Proximal phalanx

Tendon of the lateral digital extensor m.

Middle phalanx

1 - Tendon of the interosseous m. of digit IV. **2** - Proximal interphalangeal joint **3** - Base of the proximal phalanx **4** - Dorsal ligaments **5** - Dorsal sesamoid bone **6** - Head of the metacarpal bone IV **7** - Joint capsule.

Separation of the above mentioned tendons allows access to most of the proximal phalanx. Middle and distal phalanges are exposed by retraction of the tendons and ligaments that cover them.

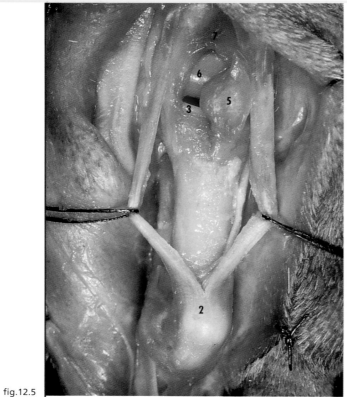

fig.12.5

After incision of the articular capsule, the articular surfaces may be seen. The dorsal sesamoid bone is very closely related to the joint (see key to fig. 12.4).

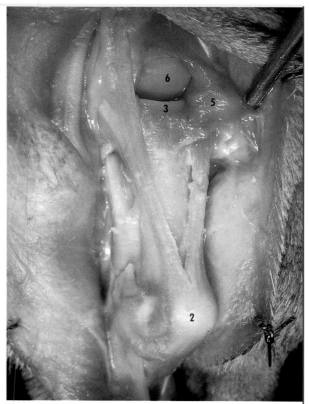

fig.12.6

Medial retraction of the dorsal sesamoid bone exposes the head of metacarpal IV and the base of the proximal phalanx of digit IV (see key to fig. 12.4).

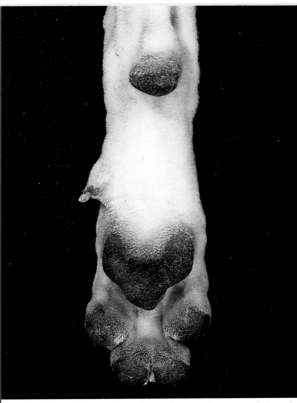

fig.13.1

The animal is in sternal or dorsal recumbency. Palmar view of the right thoracic paw.

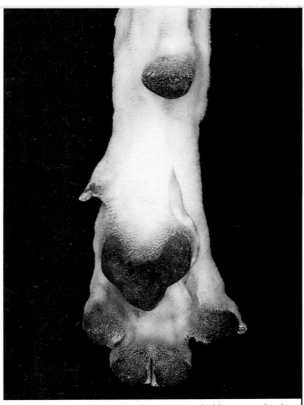

fig.13.2

The sesamoid bones of digits IV and V are approached by incising the skin laterally to the metacarpal pad. (The medial side would be the approach for the sesamoid bones of digits II and III).

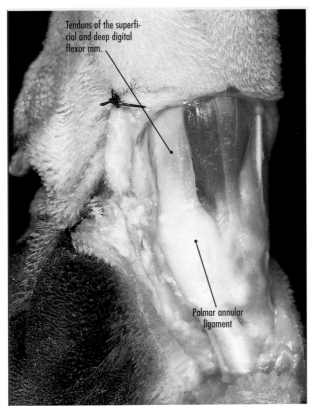

Tendons of the superficial and deep digital flexor mm.

Palmar annular ligament

fig.13.3

Palmolateral view. The subcutaneous tissues and superficial fascia are incised in the same fashion, allowing visualisation of the tendons of the superficial and deep digital flexor muscles.

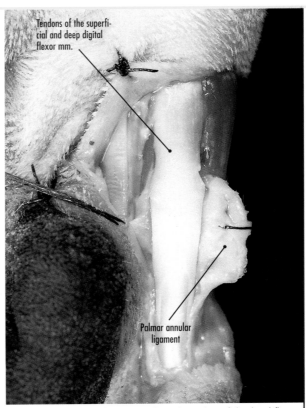

Tendons of the superficial and deep digital flexor mm.

Palmar annular ligament

fig.13.4

Next, the palmar annular ligament overlying the tendons of the digital flexor muscles is cut at the level of the metacarpophalangeal joint, allowing retraction of the tendons.

THORACIC LIMB

13

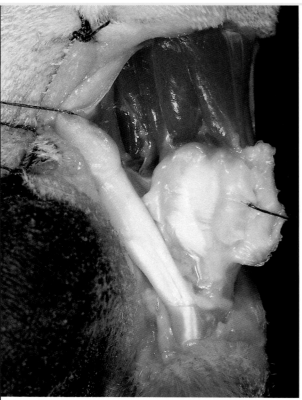

fig.13.5

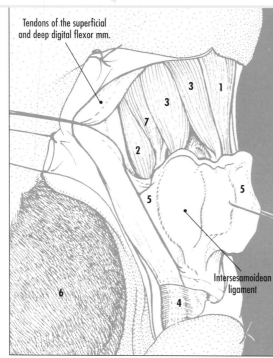

1 - Abductor digiti quinti m. 2 - Interosseous m. of digit IV. 3 - Interosseous m. of digit V
4 - Proximal digital annular ligament. 5 - Palmar annular ligament 6 - Metacarpal pad 7 - Adductor
digiti quinti m.

The medial retraction of the flexor tendons exposes the palmar aspect of the proximal sesamoid bones, covered by the intersesamoidean ligament.

The same procedure is used to approach the proximal sesamoid bones of the pelvic limb.

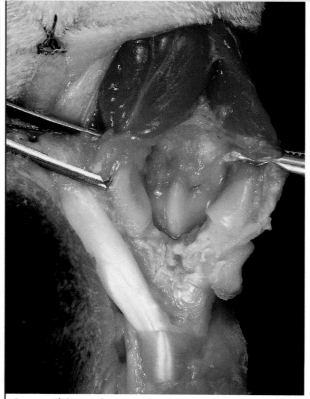

fig.13.6

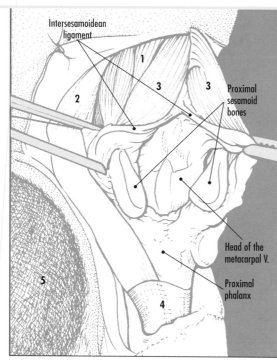

1 - Adductor digiti quinti m. 2 - Tendons of superficial and deep digital flexor Mm. 3 - Interosseous m.
of the digit V 4 - Proximal digital annular ligament. 5 - Metacarpal pad

Exposure of the articular aspect of each sesamoid bone and the palmar aspect of the head of the metacarpal bone occurs after incising the intersesamoidean ligament.

PELVIC
Limb

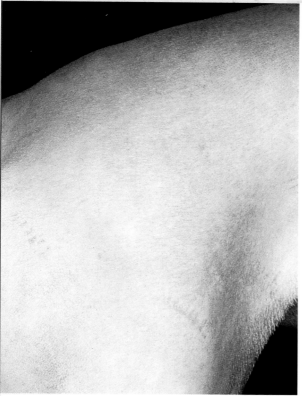

fig.14.1

The animal is in left lateral recumbency. Lateral view of the right pelvic limb.

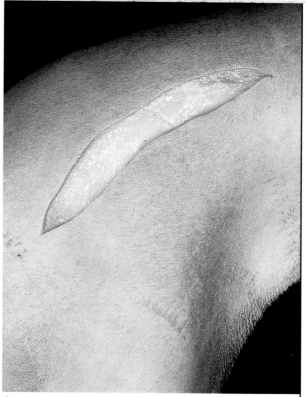

fig.14.2

The cutaneous incision extends from the centre of the iliac crest to a site located just caudal and distal to the greater trochanter of the femur. These bony landmarks are easily palpable.

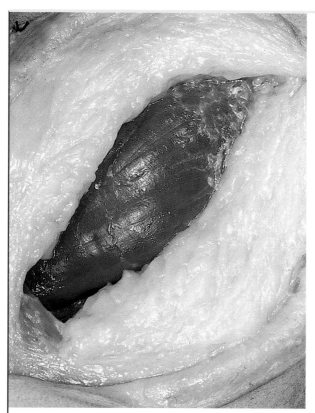

fig.14.3

An incision in the same direction as the previous one, is made through the subcutaneous tissue, which is usually quite fatty, and the gluteal fascia. This permits better visualisation of the middle gluteal muscle.

Middle gluteal m.

Tensor fasciae latae m.

1

1 - Biceps femoris m.

14

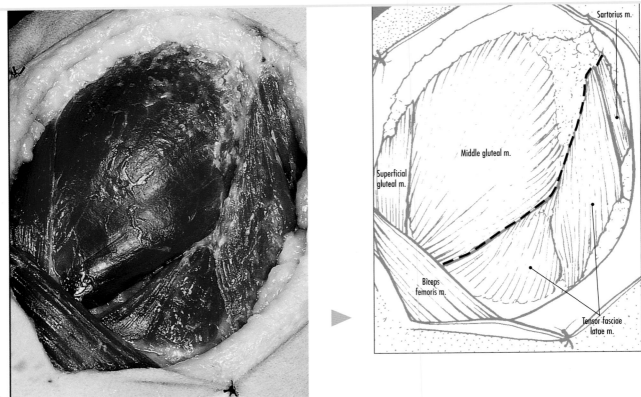

fig.14.4

The next step is separation of the middle gluteal muscle from both parts of the tensor fasciae latae muscle, from the iliac crest to the cranial border of the biceps femoris muscle. In addition, the origin of the middle gluteal muscle is incised over the length of the ventral border of the wing of the ilium; the incision is extended dorsally to allow adequate retraction of the above-mentioned muscle. The photo shows the area of interest, after most of the gluteal fascia has been removed, in order to facilitate identification of the different structures.

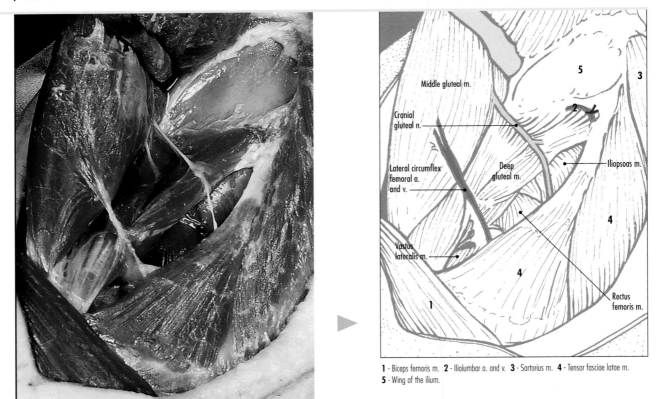

1 - Biceps femoris m. 2 - Iliolumbar a. and v. 3 - Sartorius m. 4 - Tensor fasciae latae m.
5 - Wing of the ilium.

fig.14.5

Dorsal retraction of the middle gluteal muscle shows the majority of the wing of the ilium and the deep gluteal muscle. The iliolumbar vessels are generally ligated.

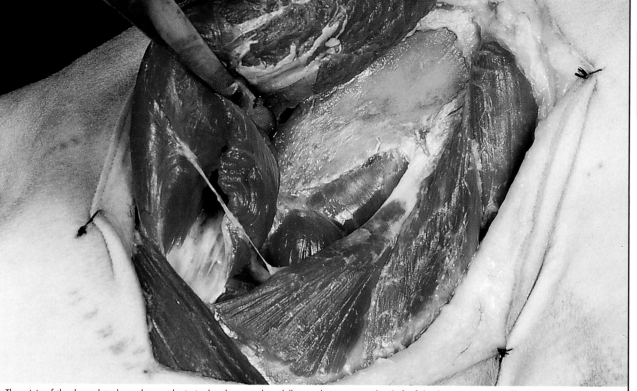

The ventral retraction of the iliopsoas muscle involves sectioning the nutrient artery of the bone that must then be thermocoagulated or ligated.

fig.14.6

The origin of the deep gluteal muscle must be incised and retracted caudally in order to expose the shaft of the ilium. Despite the efforts to preserve the cranial gluteal nerve that goes to the tensor fasciae latae muscle, it is sometimes sectioned but without clinical repercussions.

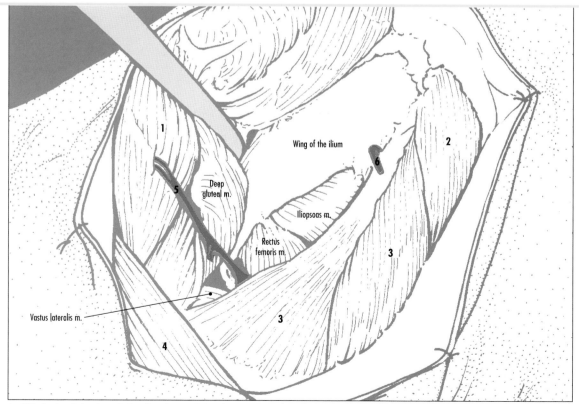

Wing of the ilium

Deep gluteal m.

Iliopsoas m.

Rectus femoris m.

Vastus lateralis m.

1 - Middle gluteal m.   **2** - Sartorius m.   **3** - Tensor fasciae latae m.   **4** - Biceps femoris m.   **5** - Lateral circumflex femoral a. and v.   **6** - Iliolumbar a. and v.

Craniodorsal Approach to the Hip Joint

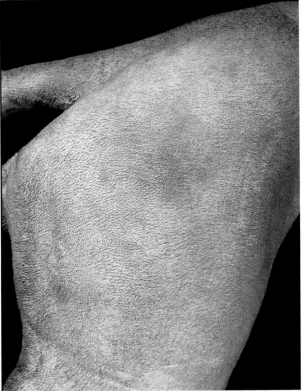

fig.15.1

The animal is in left lateral recumbency. Lateral view of the right pelvic limb.

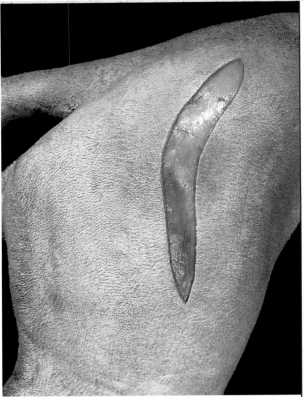

fig.15.2

The cutaneous incision may either run straight from the dorsal midline, above the greater trochanter and extend distally to the proximal third of the femoral shaft, or, as in the photo, a dorsocranially curved incision over the gluteal area.

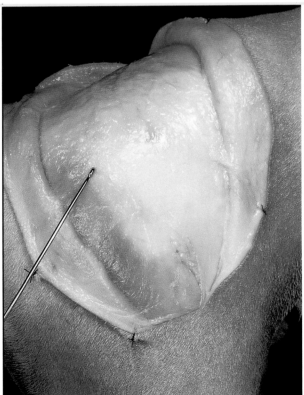

fig.15.3

Palpation of the greater trochanter helps to locate where to incise the subcutaneous tissue, generally infiltrated with fat.

Biceps femoris m.

1 - Greater trochanter of the femur

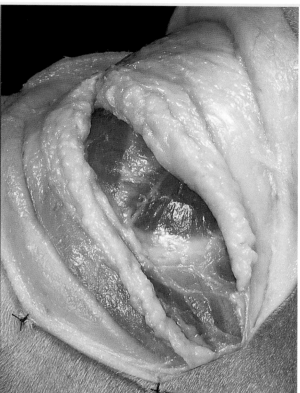

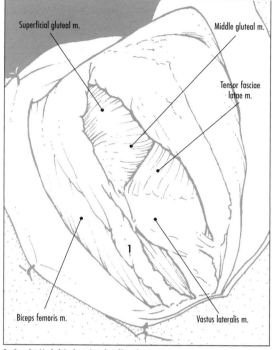

1 - Superficial leaf of the fascia lata, fat infiltrated.

fig.15.4

The subcutaneous incision is straight and slightly cranial to the greater trochanter. The superficial leaf of the fascia lata is incised along the cranial border of the biceps femoris muscle.

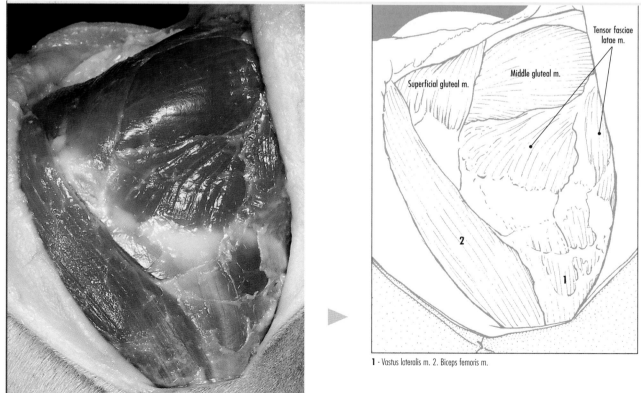

1 - Vastus lateralis m. 2. Biceps femoris m.

fig.15.5

The next step is separation of the tensor fasciae latae, middle gluteal and superficial gluteal muscles. The image shows the area after most of the deep fascia has been retracted to improve the visualisation of the various structures.

15

Partial incision of the deep leaf of the fascia lata allows cranioventral retraction of the tensor fasciae latae muscle, enlarging the approach (dotted line).

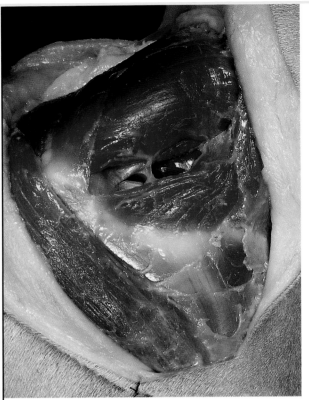

fig.15.6

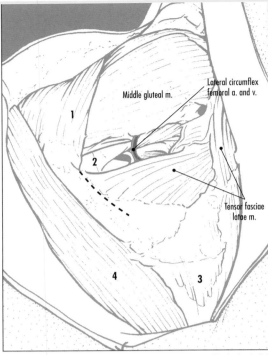

Middle gluteal m.

Lateral circumflex femoral a. and v.

Tensor fasciae latae m.

1 - Superficial gluteal m. 2 - Deep gluteal m. 3 - Vastus lateralis m. (covered by the deep leaf of the fascia lata) 4 - Biceps femoris m.

Dissecting between the middle gluteal and tensor fasciae latae muscles generally results in damage to the lateral circumflex femoral vessels.

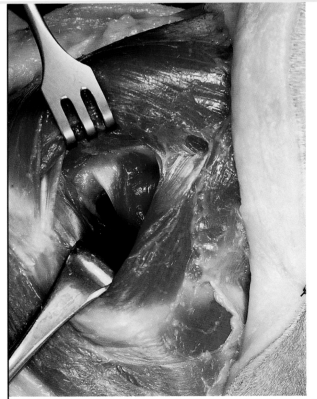

fig.15.7

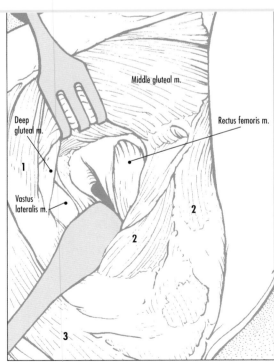

Middle gluteal m.

Deep gluteal m.

Rectus femoris m.

Vastus lateralis m.

1 - Superficial gluteal m. 2 - Tensor fasciae latae m. 3 - Biceps femoris m

Blunt dissection and separation on the neck of the femur with the fingertips allows visualisation of the classic triangle bounded dorsally by the middle and deep gluteal muscles, craniomedially by the rectus femoris muscle and caudolaterally by the vastus lateralis muscle.

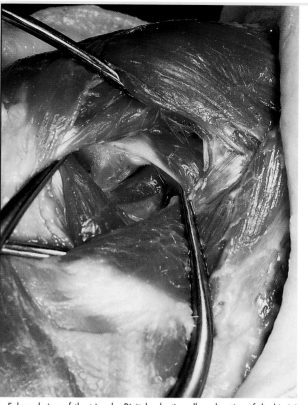

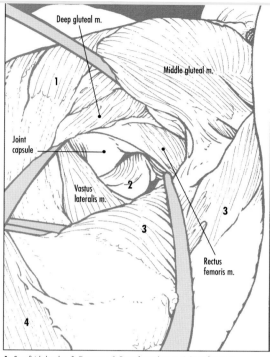

1 - Superficial gluteal m. 2. Iliopsoas m. 3. Tensor fasciae latae m. 4. Biceps femoris m.

fig.15.8

Enlarged view of the triangle. Digital palpation allows location of the hip joint while the limb is being manipulated.

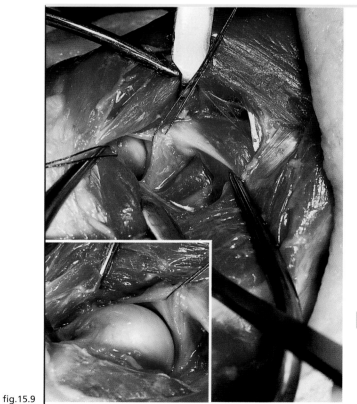

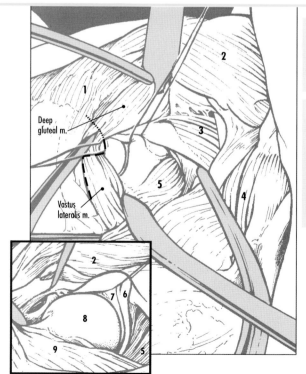

Positioning surgical retractors on the medial aspect of the body of the ilium must be done with care to avoid injury to the sciatic nerve.

Partial tenomyotomy of the deep gluteal muscle (dotted line) improves the visualisation of the acetabular rim, while partial tenomyotomy of the vastus lateralis muscle improves the visualisation of the femoral neck (broken line).

1 - Superficial gluteal m. **2** - Middle gluteal m. **3** - Rectus femoris m. **4** - Tensor fasciae latae m.
5 - Iliopsoas m. **6** - Joint capsule **7** - Acetabular rim **8** - Femoral head **9** - Vastus lateralis m.

fig.15.9

Arthrotomy reveals the femoral head and acetabulum.

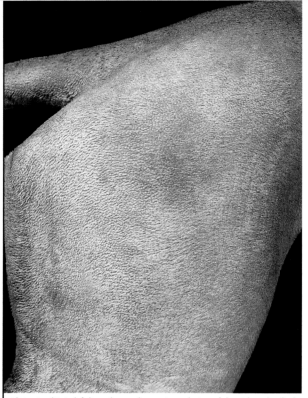

fig.16.1

The animal is in left lateral recumbency. Lateral view of the right pelvic limb.

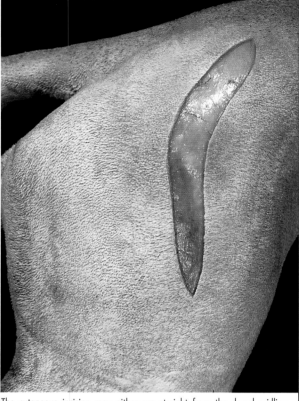

fig.16.2

The cutaneous incision may either run straight from the dorsal midline, above the greater trochanter and extend distally to the proximal third of the femoral shaft; or, as in the photo, a dorsocranially curved incision over the gluteal area.

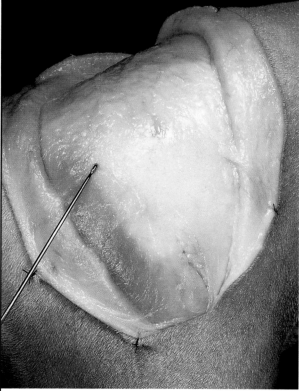

fig.16.3

Palpation of the greater trochanter helps to locate where to incise the subcutaneous tissue, generally infiltrated with fat (see fig. 15.3).

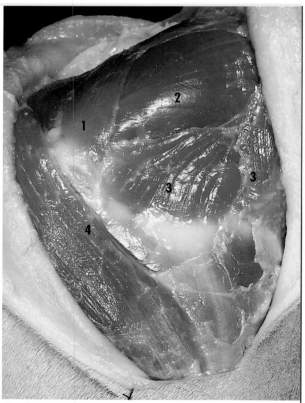

fig.16.4

The subcutaneous tissue is incised in a straight line, just cranial to the greater trochanter (see fig.15.4) revealing the superficial gluteal (**1**), middle gluteal (**2**), tensor fasciae latae (**3**) and biceps femoris (**4**) muscles.

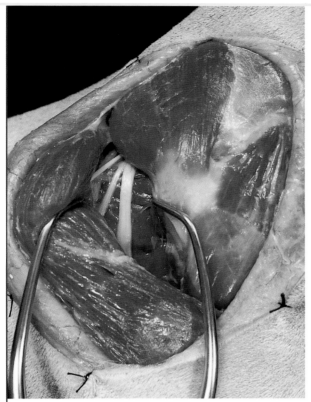

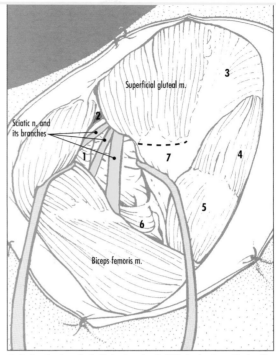

1 - Quadratus femoris m. 2 - Caudal gluteal a. and v. 3 - Middle gluteal m. (covered by gluteal fascia) 4 - Tensor fasciae latae m. 5 - Vastus lateralis m. (covered by fascia lata) 6 - Adductor m. 7 - Greater trochanter.

fig.16.5

The biceps femoris muscle is retracted caudally, exposing the sciatic nerve and its muscular branches. The insertion of the superficial gluteal muscle is incised, being careful to leave enough tendon at the trochanteric level to permit subsequent repair.

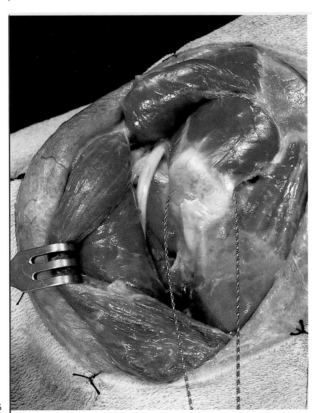

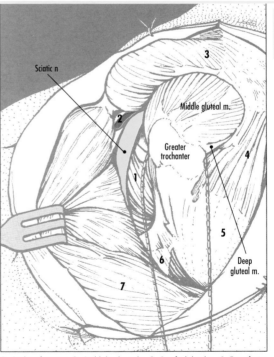

The separated trochanter is reattached to the femur by a tension band device.

1 - Quadratus femoris m. 2 - Caudal gluteal a. and v. 3 - Superficial gluteal m. 4 - Tensor fasciae latae m. 5 - Vastus lateralis m. 6 - Adductor m. 7 - Biceps femoris m.

fig.16.6

The insertions of the middle gluteal, deep gluteal and piriformis muscles to the greater trochanter are exposed by dorsally retracting the superficial gluteal muscle. A Gigli wire is used to cut through the greater trochanter underneath the tendons of the above-mentioned muscles. The sciatic nerve must be protected during the osteotomy. The osteotomy can also be performed using a chisel or oscillating saw. The osteotomy is carried out at a 45° angle to the long axis of the femur.

PELVIC LIMB

16

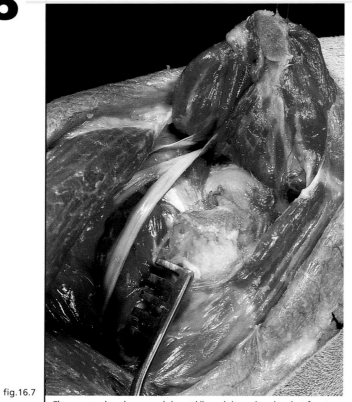

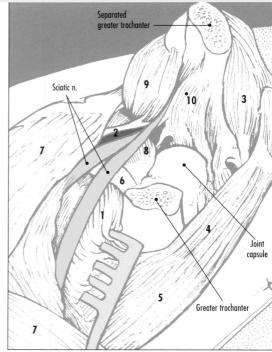

1 - Quadratus femoris m. **2** - Caudal gluteal a. and v. **3** - Middle gluteal m. **4** - Tensor fasciae latae m. **5** - Vastus lateralis m. **6** - Internal obturator m. **7** - Biceps femoris m. **8** - Cranial gemellus m. **9** - Piriformis m. **10** - Deep gluteal m.

fig.16.7

The separated trochanter and the middle and deep gluteal and piriformis muscles are retracted craniodorsally, exposing the articular capsule.

The approach can be enlarged caudally by tenotomy of the gemelli and internal obturator muscles (broken line); and cranially by periosteal elevation of the deep gluteal muscle (dotted line).

Complete tenotomy of the gluteal muscles is the alternative to this approach. The tendons must be re-attached to the greater trochanter by anchoring the sutures through holes made in its base.

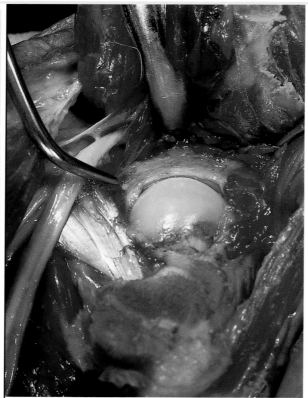

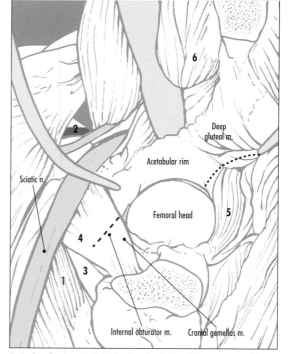

1 - Quadratus femoris m. **2** - Caudal gluteal a. and v. **3** - External obturator m. **4** - Caudal gemellus m. **5** - Articularis coxae m. **6** - Middle gluteal m.

fig.16.8

Arthrotomy exposes the femoral head and the dorsal acetabular rim.

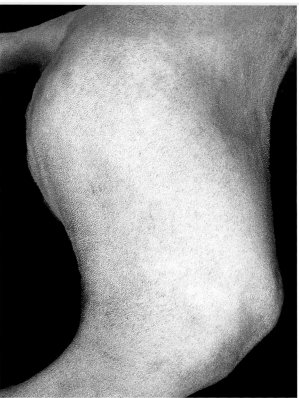

fig.17.1

The animal is in left lateral recumbency. Lateral view of the right pelvic limb.

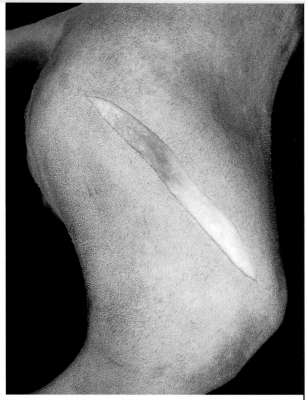

fig.17.2

The cutaneous incision extends from the greater trochanter to the lateral epicondyle of the femur.

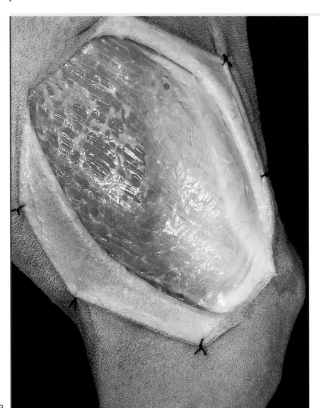

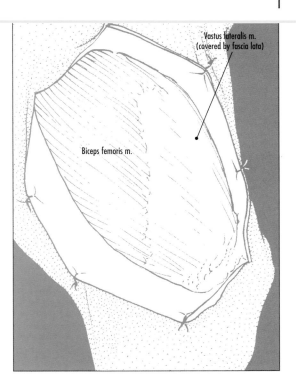

Vastus lateralis m.
(covered by fascia lata)

Biceps femoris m.

fig.17.3

The fascia lata is exposed by retraction of the subcutaneous tissue. It covers the vastus lateralis muscle and is also the insertion of the biceps femoris muscle.

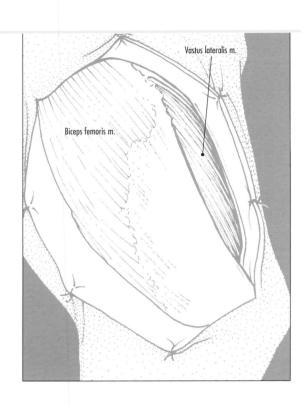

fig.17.4

The fascia lata is incised following the direction of the femoral shaft, a few centimetres cranial to the biceps femoris muscle.

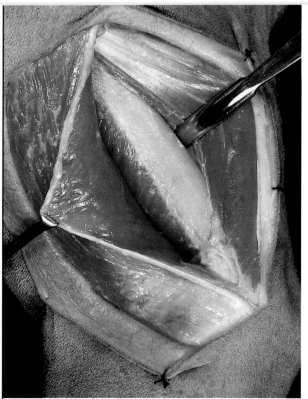

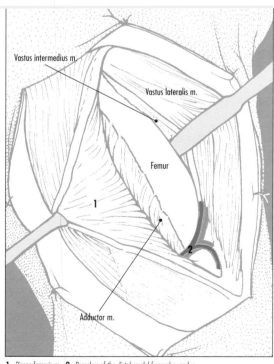

1 - Biceps femoris m.   2 - Branches of the distal caudal femoral a. and v.

fig.17.5

The femoral shaft is exposed by caudal retraction of the biceps femoris muscle and cranial retraction of the vastus lateralis and vastus intermedius muscles.

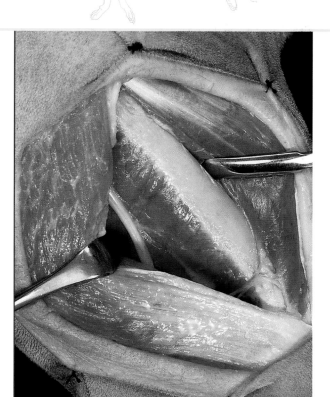

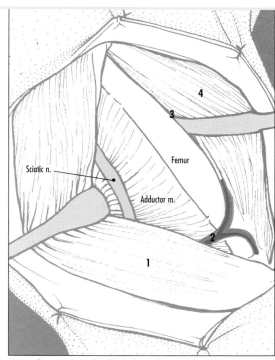

1 - Biceps femoris m. **2** - Branches of the distal caudal femoral a. and v. **3** - Vastus intermedius m.
4 - Vastus lateralis m.

fig.17.6

The sciatic nerve is located on the adductor muscle a few centimetres caudal to the femoral shaft.

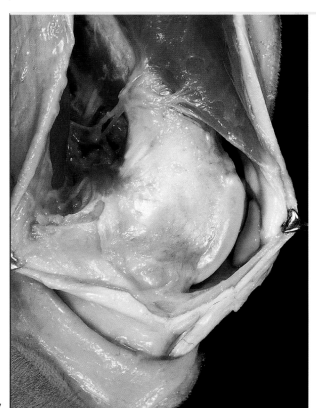

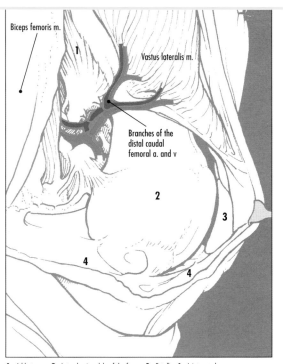

1 - Adductor m. **2** - Lateral epicondyle of the femur **3** - Patella **4** - Joint capsule

fig.17.7

The approach can be enlarged distally by extending the incision of the fascia lata and separating the vastus lateralis and biceps femoris muscles. If necessary, the muscular branches of the distal caudal femoral vessels can be sectioned to gain better access to the supracondylar area of the femur. In this view, the articular capsule of the stifle joint has been incised to improve the visualisation of the anatomical structures.

Lateral Approach to the Stifle

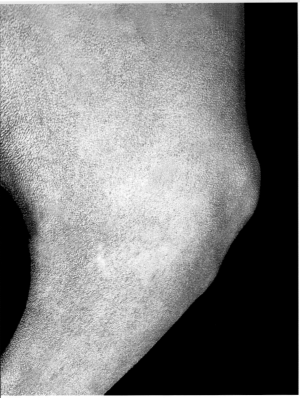

fig.18.1

The animal is in left lateral recumbency. Lateral view of the right pelvic limb.

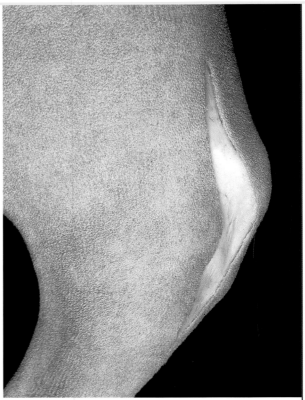

fig.18.2

A parapatellar curved cutaneous incision extends from the distal third of the femur to the tibial tuberosity.

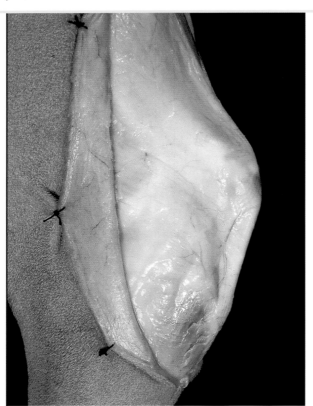

fig.18.3

Fascia lata

Patellar ligament

Fascia of the stifle joint

Cranial tibial m.

Retraction of the subcutaneous tissue exposes the distal fascia lata and the stifle fascia. These two fascias and the joint capsule are incised in the same parapatellar fashion, ensuring enough tissue is left on the patellar area to be able to close the joint. A stab incision is made with the blade into the capsule just lateral to the patellar ligament, and enlarged with scissors proximally and distally, to avoid damaging the femoral articular cartilage.

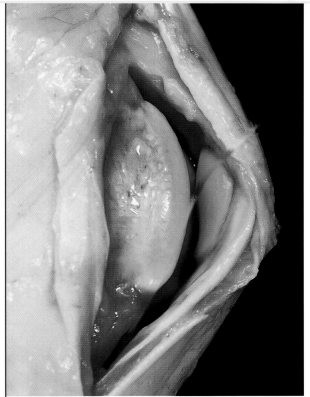

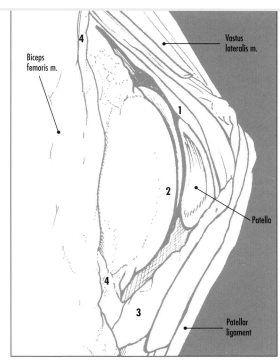

1 - Lateral parapatellar fibrocartilage 2 - Femoral trochlea 3 - Infrapatellar fat body 4 - Joint capsule

fig.18.4

The patella is luxated medially in the extended joint, once arthrotomy has been performed. It is often necessary to incise between the biceps femoris and vastus lateralis muscles. The distal caudal femoral vessels should be ligated at this point (see fig. 17.7)

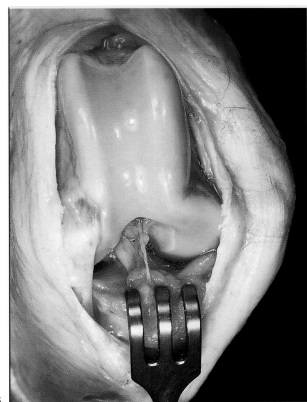

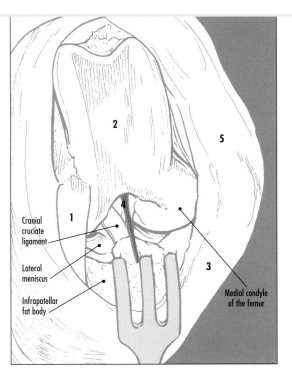

1 - Tendon of the long digital extensor m. 2 - Femoral trochlea 3 - Patellar ligament 4 - Intra-articular vessels 5 - Displaced patella.

fig.18.5

Cranial view of the right stifle showing the articular surface of the femoral condyles and the cranial portion of the menisci once the patella and the infrapatellar fat body have been retracted distally. There is a small blood vessel cranial to the cruciate ligaments.

18

In order to visualise the caudal pole of the menisci, a Hoffmann retractor is placed intra-articularly to distract the femoral and tibial articular surfaces.

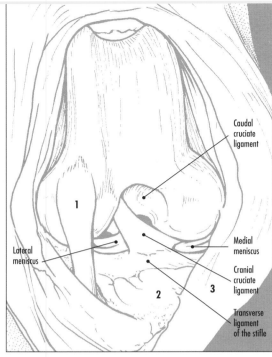

Caudal cruciate ligament

Lateral meniscus

Medial meniscus

Cranial cruciate ligament

Transverse ligament of the stifle

1 - Tendon of the long digital extensor m. **2** - Infrapatellar fat body **3** - Patellar ligament

fig.18.6

Stifle hyperflexion allows inspection of the cruciate ligaments. Removal of the infrapatellar fat body reveals the anterior aspect of the menisci and the transverse ligament of the stifle (intermeniscal ligament).

APPENDIX

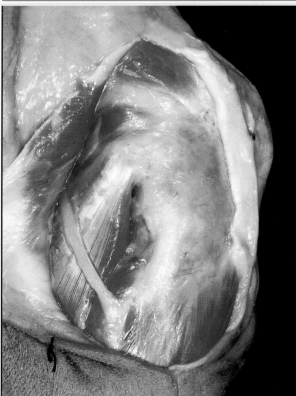

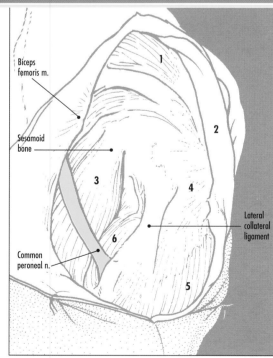

Biceps femoris m.

Sesamoid bone

Common peroneal n.

Lateral collateral ligament

1 - Vastus lateralis m. **2** - Retracted fascia **3** - Gastrocnemius m. (lateral head) **4** - Joint capsule **5** - Tibialis cranialis m. **6** - Popliteus m.

fig.18.7

Anatomical dissection of the lateral stifle showing the common peroneal nerve, the collateral ligament and the sesamoid bone of the gastrocnemius muscle (lateral head). This view is achieved after incising the fascia and retracting caudally the biceps femoris muscle.

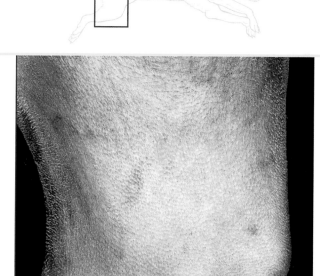

fig.19.1

The animal is in left lateral recumbency. Medial view of the left pelvic limb.

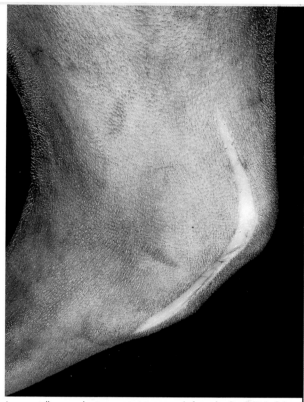

fig.19.2

A parapatellar curved cutaneous incision extends from the distal third of the femur to the tibial tuberosity.

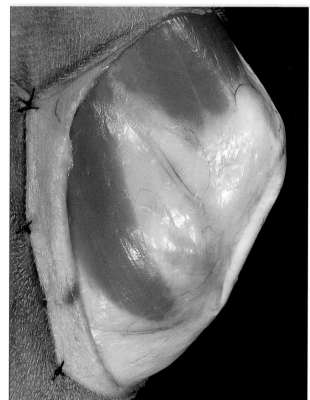

fig.19.3

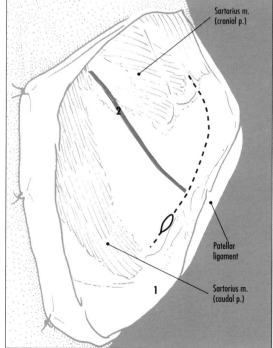

Sartorius m. (cranial p.)

2

Patellar ligament

Sartorius m. (caudal p.)

1

1 -Tibial tuberosity **2** -Descending genicular a. and v.

Arthrotomy is performed by a stab incision with a scalpel, medial to the patellar ligament. The incision is extended by scissors, reaching the distal portion of the vastus medialis muscle. Enough tissue is left to allow closure of the joint.

19

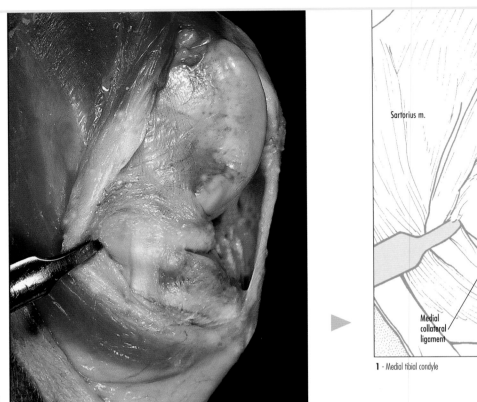

1 - Medial tibial condyle

fig.19.4

The caudal retraction of the joint capsule exposes the articular structures. The arthrotomy is extended proximally until the patella can be luxated laterally.

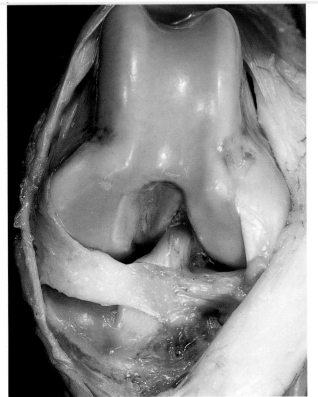

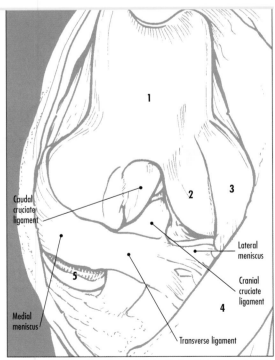

1 - Femoral trochlea 2 - Lateral femoral condyle 3 - Tendon of the long digital extensor m. 4 - Patellar ligament 5 - Medial tibial condyle

fig.19.5

Cranial view of the left stifle. Stifle hyperflexion with the patella luxated laterally allows inspection of the cruciate ligaments. Removal of the infrapatellar fat body reveals the anterior aspect of the menisci and the transverse ligament of the stifle (intermeniscal ligament).

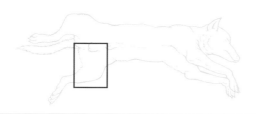

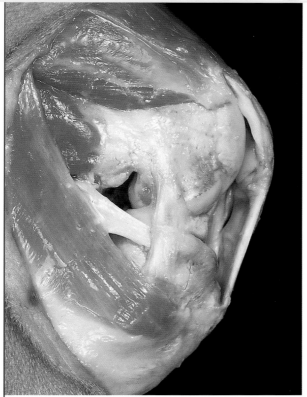

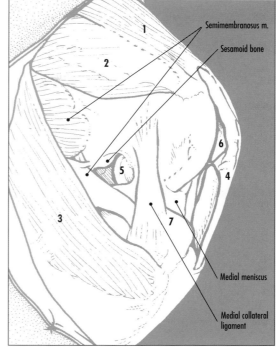

Semimembranosus m.

Sesamoid bone

1 - Sartorius m. (cranial p.) 2 - Vastus medialis m. 3 - Sartorius m. (caudal p.) 4 - Patellar ligament
5 - Medial femoral condyle 6 - Patella 7 - Medial tibial condyle

Medial meniscus

Medial collateral ligament

fig.19.6

Anatomical dissection of the medial region of the stifle, showing the intimate relationship between the medial collateral ligament and the medial meniscus. One can also see the double insertion of the semimembranous muscle, and the sesamoid bone of the gastrocnemius muscle (medial head).

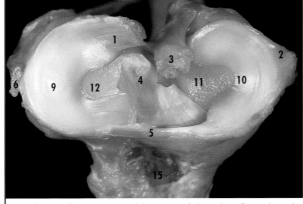

fig.19.7

Dorsal view of the menisci and ligaments of the right stifle, without the femur.

Key to figs. 19.7 and 19.8

1	Femoral ligament of the lateral meniscus	**9**	Lateral meniscus
2	Medial collateral ligament	**10**	Medial meniscus
3	Caudal cruciate ligament	**11**	Medial tibial condyle
4	Cranial cruciate ligament	**12**	Lateral tibial condyle
5	Transverse ligament	**13**	Medial femoral condyle
6	Lateral collateral ligament	**14**	Lateral femoral condyle
7	Tibial insertion of the lateral meniscus	**15**	Tibial tuberosity
		16	Sesamoid bones of the gastrocnemius m.
8	Tendon of the popliteus m.	**17**	Fibula.

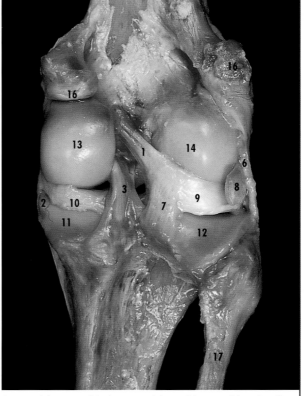

fig.19.8

Anatomical dissection of the ligaments of the caudal aspect of the right stifle.

Medial Approach
to the Shaft of the Tibia

20

The cutaneous incision is curved cranially if a bone plate is going to be used in the repair, avoiding contact of the bone plate with the surgical wound.

The medial saphenous vein is raised to improve its visualisation, to avoid cutting into it during the skin incision.

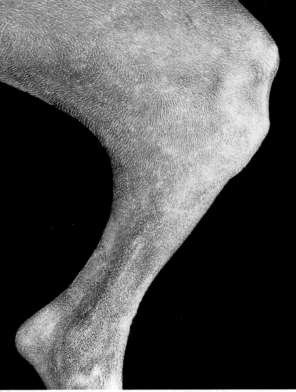

fig.20.1

The animal is in left lateral recumbency. Medial view of the left pelvic limb.

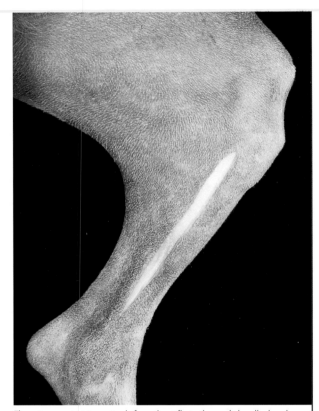

fig.20.2

The cutaneous incision extends from the stifle to the medial malleolus along the area of palpation of the tibial shaft.

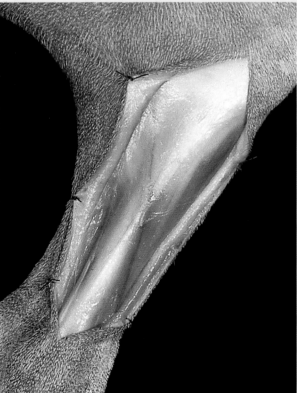

fig.20.3

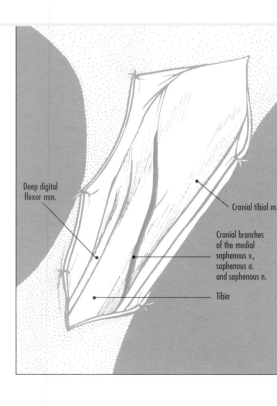

Deep digital flexor mm.

Cranial tibial m.

Cranial branches of the medial saphenous v., saphenous a. and saphenous n.

Tibia

The subcutaneous tissue dissection exposes the cranial branch of the medial saphenous vein, together with the cranial branch of the saphenous artery and the saphenous nerve. These structures cross the tibial shaft at its middle third.

PELVIC LIMB

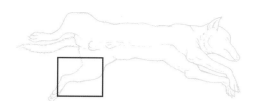

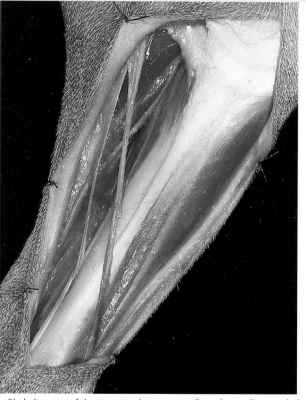

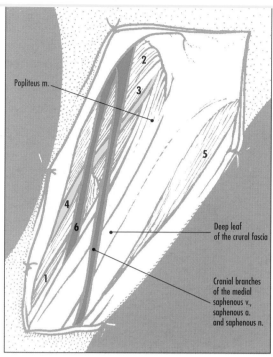

Popliteus m.

Deep leaf
of the crural fascia

Cranial branches
of the medial
saphenous v.,
saphenous a.
and saphenous n.

1 - Deep digital flexor mm. **2** - Gastrocnemius m. (medial head) **3** - Superficial digital flexor m.
4 - Tibial n. **5** - Tibialis cranialis m. **6** - Caudal branches of the medial saphenous v., saphenous a. and saphenous n.

fig.20.4

Block dissection of the neurovascular structures allows them to be moved, thereby improving the surgical approach.

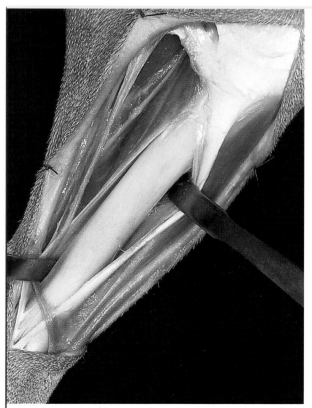

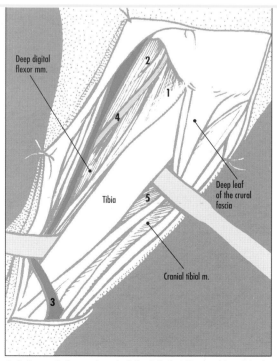

Deep digital
flexor mm.

Tibia

Deep leaf
of the crural
fascia

Cranial tibial m.

1 - Popliteus m. **2** - Gastrocnemius m. (medial head) **3** - Cranial branches of the medial saphenous v., saphenous a. and saphenous n. **4** - Tibial n. **5** - Long digital extensor m.

fig.20.5

Most of the tibial shaft is exposed by incising the crural fascia, together with the lateral retraction of the tibialis cranialis muscle and long digital extensor muscle, cranial retraction of the deep leaf of the crural fascia, and caudal retraction of the deep digital flexor muscles.

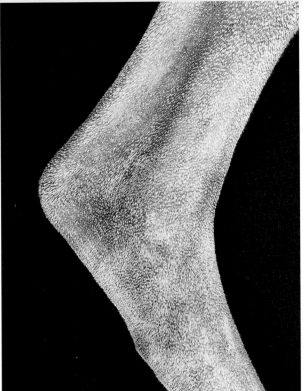

fig.21.1

The animal is in left lateral recumbency. Medial view of the left pelvic limb.

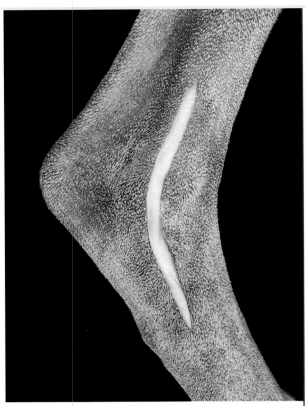

fig.21.2

The curved cutaneous incision is centred on the medial malleolus, starting in the distal third of the tibia and finishing at the tarsometatarsal joint.

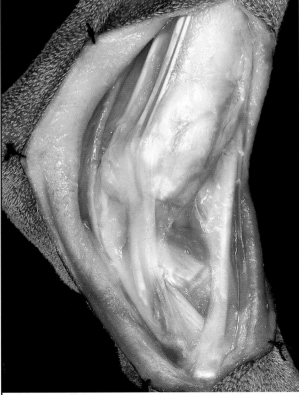

fig.21.3

After the subcutaneous tissues have been dissected, the medial collateral ligament and the tendon of the tibialis cranialis muscle are exposed. Arthrotomy of the talocrural joint will be performed cranially and caudally to the medial collateral ligament.

Flexor retinaculum

Medial collateral ligament (long p.)

Medial malleolus

Tendon of the tibialis cranialis m.

See key on page 83

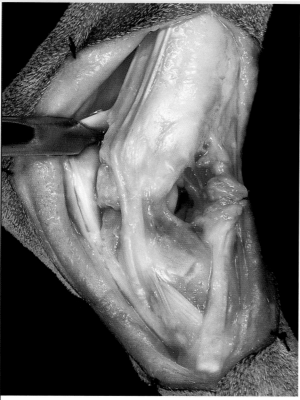

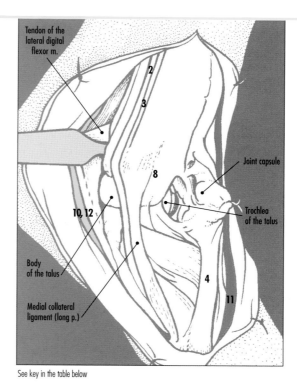

Tendon of the
lateral digital
flexor m.

2

3

8

Joint capsule

10, 12

Trochlea
of the talus

Body
of the talus

Medial collateral
ligament (long p.)

4

11

See key in the table below

fig.21.4

The longitudinal incision to both sides of the medial collateral ligament allows access to the dorsal and plantar aspects of the talocrural joint. The caudal incision cuts the flexor retinaculum, freeing the tendon of the lateral digital flexor muscle.

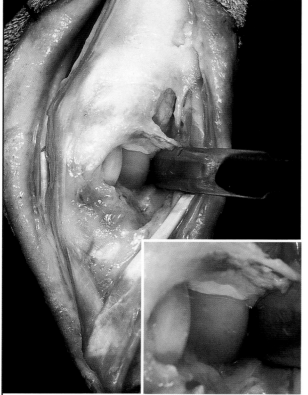

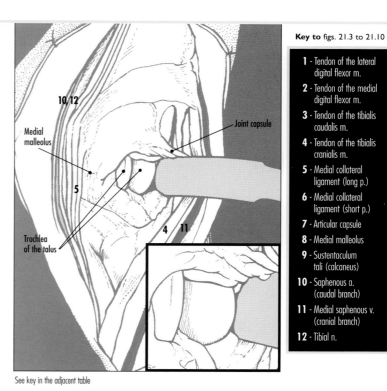

10, 12

Medial
malleolus

Joint capsule

5

4   11

Trochlea
of the talus

Key to figs. 21.3 to 21.10

1 - Tendon of the lateral
digital flexor m.

2 - Tendon of the medial
digital flexor m.

3 - Tendon of the tibialis
caudalis m.

4 - Tendon of the tibialis
cranialis m.

5 - Medial collateral
ligament (long p.)

6 - Medial collateral
ligament (short p.)

7 - Articular capsule

8 - Medial malleolus

9 - Sustentaculum
tali (calcaneus)

10 - Saphenous a.
(caudal branch)

11 - Medial saphenous v.
(cranial branch)

12 - Tibial n.

See key in the adjacent table

fig.21.5

Dorsomedial view of the tarsus. The trochlea of the talus is visualised after retracting the joint capsule dorsolaterally whilst extending the joint.

21

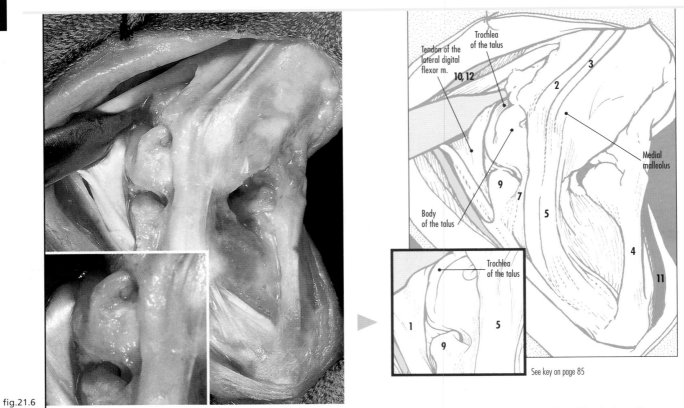

Tendon of the
lateral digital
flexor m.

Trochlea
of the talus

10, 12

3

2

Medial
malleolus

9

7

5

Body
of the talus

Trochlea
of the talus

1

5

9

4

11

See key on page 85

fig.21.6

Plantar retraction of the tendon of the lateral digital flexor muscle while the joint is flexed, reveals the posterior aspect of the trochlea of the tibial tarsal bone.

OSTEOTOMY OF THE MEDIAL MALLEOLUS

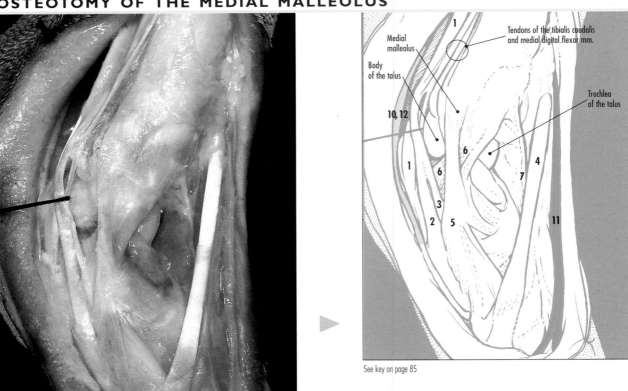

1

Tendons of the tibialis caudalis
and medial digital flexor mm.

Medial
malleolus

Body
of the talus

10, 12

1

6

6

3

2

5

Trochlea
of the talus

6

7

4

11

See key on page 85

fig.21.7

Incision of the flexor retinaculum frees the tendons of the tibialis caudalis and the medial digital flexor muscles from the groove of the medial malleolus.

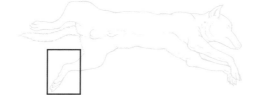

The detached fragment is fixed with a lag screw or a tension band device, avoiding entering the tibial cochlea.

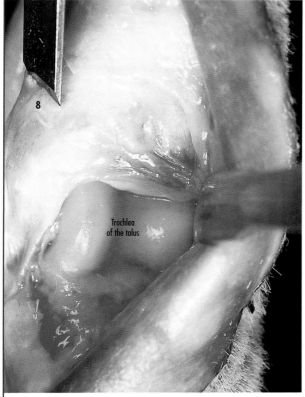

fig.21.8

The chisel is positioned at such an angle that the osteotomy plane involves most of the medial malleolus, without affecting the articular surfaces of the cochlea of the tibia and the trochlea of the tibial tarsal bone (see key to the table below).

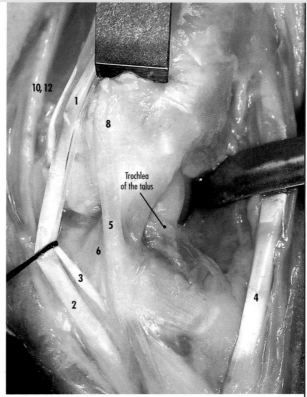

fig.21.9

The detached piece of bone includes most of the area of insertion of the medial collateral ligament (see key to the table below).

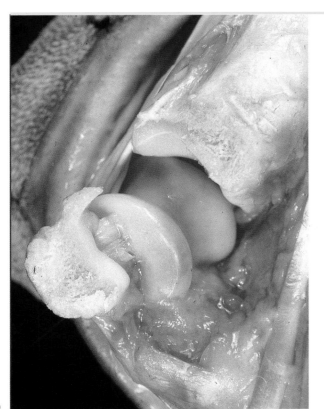

fig.21.10

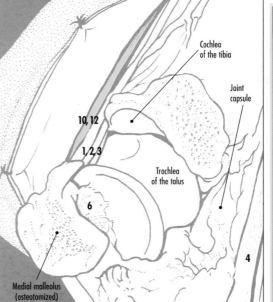

See key in the adjacent table

Most of the trochlea of the tibial tarsal bone is exposed by distal retraction of the detached malleolus, and internal rotation of the joint.

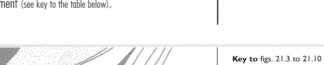

Key to figs. 21.3 to 21.10

1	- Tendon of the lateral digital flexor m.
2	- Tendon of the medial digital flexor m.
3	- Tendon of the tibialis caudalis m.
4	- Tendon of the tibialis cranialis m.
5	- Medial collateral ligament (long p.)
6	- Medial collateral ligament (short p.)
7	- Articular capsule
8	- Medial malleolus
9	- Sustentaculum tali (calcaneus)
10	- Saphenous a. (caudal branch)
11	- Medial saphenous v. (cranial branch)
12	- Tibial n.

PELVIC LIMB

22

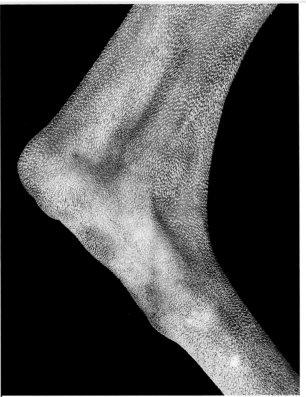

fig.22.1

The animal is in left lateral recumbency. Lateral view of the right pelvic limb.

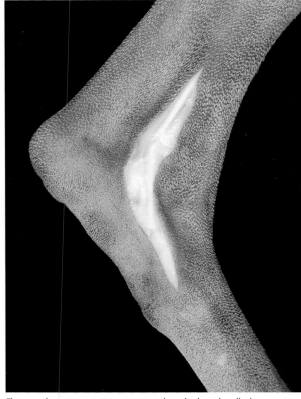

fig.22.2

The curved cutaneous incision is centered on the lateral malleolus, starting in the distal third of the tibia and finishing at the tarsometatarsal joint.

PELVIC LIMB

fig.22.3

Subcutaneous tissues are dissected in the same fashion, avoiding the caudal branch of the lateral saphenous vein.

Key to figs. 22.3 to 22.15.

1 - Tendon of the peroneus longus m.	**15** - Crural extensor retinaculum
2 - Tendon of the peroneus brevis m.	**16** - Lateral extensor retinaculum
3 - Tendon of the lateral digital extensor m.	**17** - Groove of the lateral malleolus for the peroneus longus m.
4 - Tendon of the long digital extensor m.	**18** - Joint capsule
5 - Extensor digitorum brevis m.	**19** - Tibia
6 - Abductor digiti quinti m.	**20** - Fibula
7 - Tendon of the superficial digital flexor m.	**21** - Metatarsal bone V
8 - Tendon of the lateral digital flexor m.	**22** - Calcaneus
9 - 5th interosseous m.	**23** - Fourth tarsal bone
10 - Quadratus plantae m.	**24** - Saphenous a. (caudal branch)
11 - Common calcanean tendon	**25** - Cranial tibial a.
12 - Lateral collateral ligament (long p.)	**26** - Lateral saphenous v. (caudal branch)
13 - Lateral collateral ligament (short p.)	**27** - Lateral saphenous v. (cranial branch)
14 - Tarsal extensor retinaculum	**28** - Superficial peroneal n.
	29 - Tibial n.
	30 - Deep peroneal n.

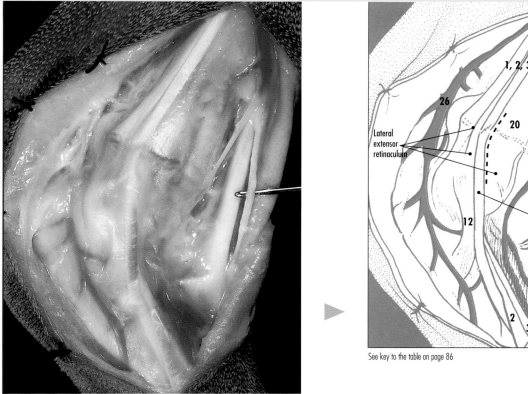

See key to the table on page 86

fig.22.4

The lateral extensor retinaculum (the retinaculum of the peroneus muscles) is identified and sectioned longitudinally along the cranial margin of the tendon of the peroneus longus muscle.

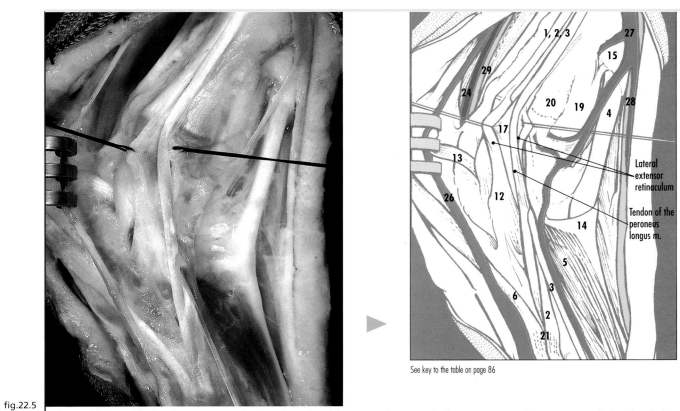

See key to the table on page 86

fig.22.5

The cranial incision of the lateral extensor retinaculum frees the tendon of the peroneus longus muscle allowing its retraction from its groove on the lateral malleolus.

22

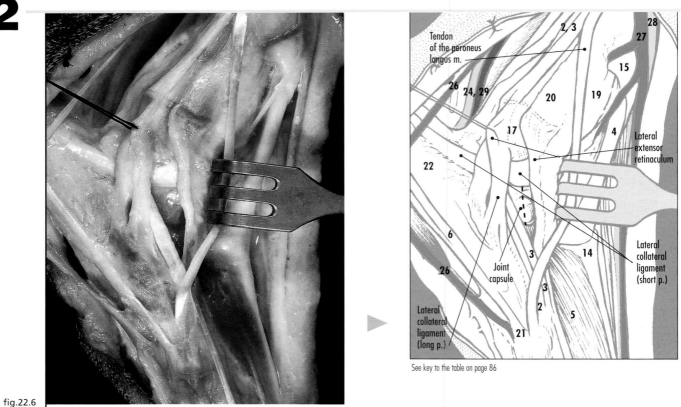

See key to the table on page 86

fig.22.6

The dorsal retraction of the tendon of the peroneus longus muscle exposes the short part of the lateral collateral ligament and joint capsule. Arthrotomy is performed parallel to the dorsal margin of the long part of the lateral collateral ligament.

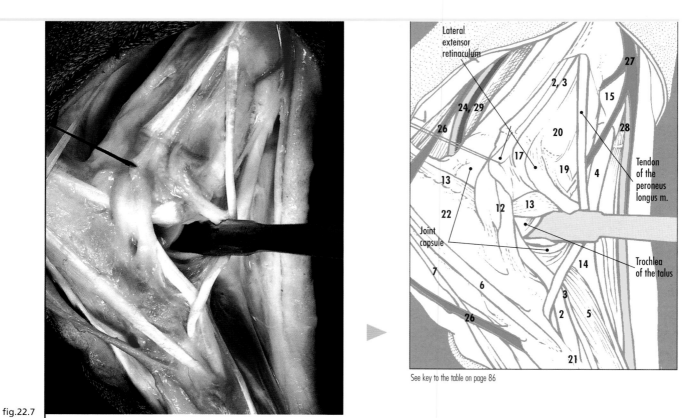

See key to the table on page 86

fig.22.7

Dorsal retraction of the articular capsule, lateral extensor retinaculum and the peroneus longus muscle exposes the dorsolateral aspect of the trochlea of the talus.

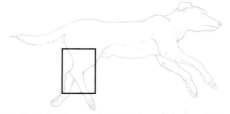

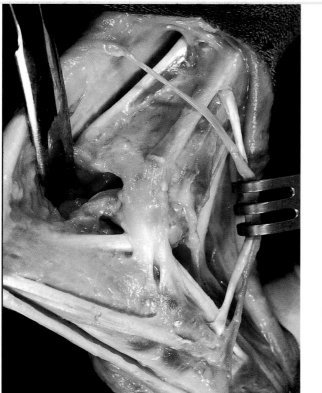

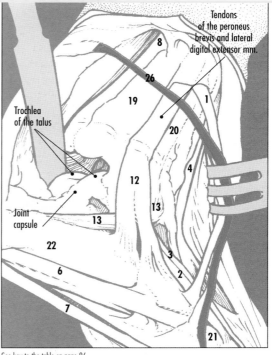

See key to the table on page 86

fig.22.8

Incision of the lateral extensor retinaculum and joint capsule, caudal to the peroneus brevis and lateral digital extensor muscles, is necessary to expose the lateroplantar aspect of the trochlea of the talus.

OSTEOTOMY OF THE LATERAL MALLEOLUS

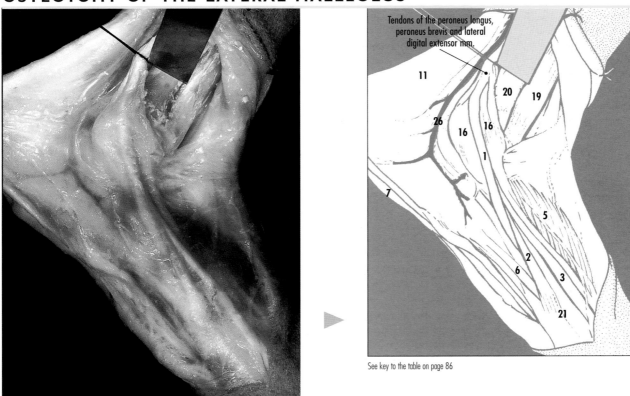

See key to the table on page 86

fig.22.9

The distal fibula is exposed by caudal retraction of the tendons of the peroneus longus, peroneus brevis and lateral digital extensor muscles. A supramalleolar osteotomy is performed, with proximal inclination. The image shows the chisel perpendicular to the fibula, in order to improve visualisation of the malleolus.

22

The separated fragment is fixed with a lag screw or tension band device, avoiding entering the tibial cochlea.

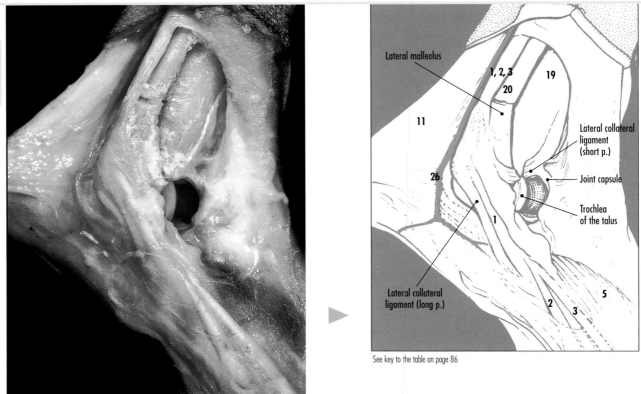

Lateral malleolus

1, 2, 3   19
20
11

Lateral collateral ligament (short p.)

26

Joint capsule

1

Trochlea of the talus

Lateral collateral ligament (long p.)

2   3   5

See key to the table on page 86

fig.22.10

The malleolus is dissected from the soft tissue attachments to the tibia, once it has been freed. Arthrotomy is performed parallel to the dorsal margin of the long part of the lateral collateral ligament. The tibial insertion of the short part of the lateral collateral ligament is incised in order to allow complete plantar separation of the lateral malleolus.

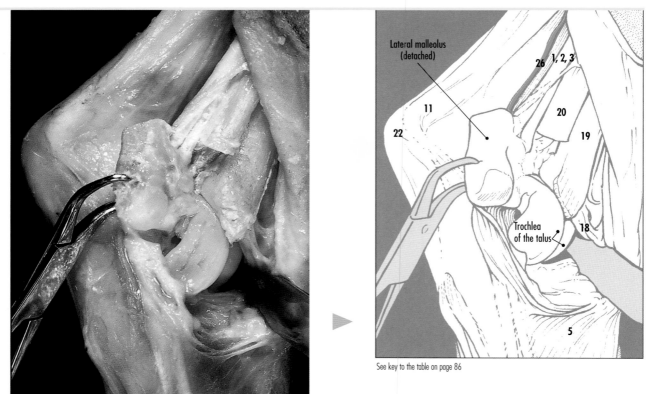

Lateral malleolus (detached)

26   1, 2, 3

11
22   20
19

Trochlea of the talus

18

5

See key to the table on page 86

fig.22.11

Plantar retraction of the malleolus exposes the talocrural joint. The cochlea of the tibia and the trochlea of the talus are exposed by extension, flexion and external rotation of the joint.

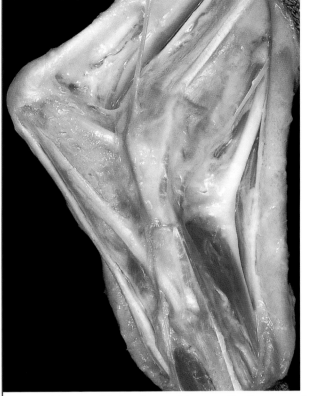

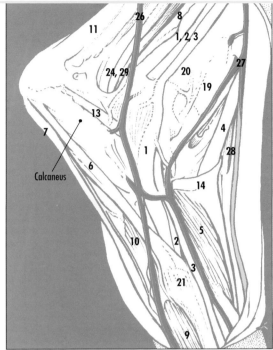

See key to the table on page 86

fig.22.12 Anatomical dissection of the lateral aspect of the tarsus. After the cutaneous incision, the fascia has been removed. The subcutaneous location of the calcaneus and the lack of neurovascular structures at this level, facilitates the lateral surgical approach to this bone.

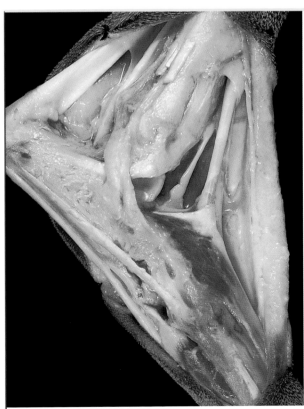

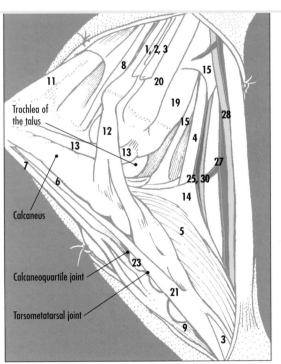

See key to the table on page 86

fig.22.13 Deep anatomical dissection of the lateral aspect of the tarsus. The tendons of the peroneus brevis, peroneus longus, lateral digital extensor muscles and the caudal branch of the lateral saphenous vein have been removed. The talocrural (talus-tibia), calcaneoquartile (calcaneus-tarsal bone IV) and tarsometatarsal joints are exposed.

PELVIC LIMB

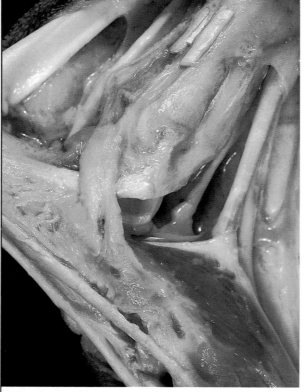

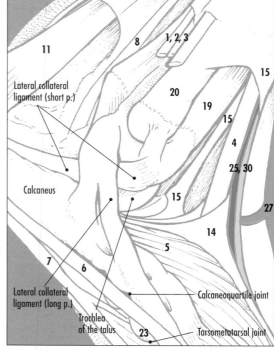

11 8 1, 2, 3
15
Lateral collateral
ligament (short p.)
20
19
15
15
4
25, 30
Calcaneus
15
27
14
5
7
6
Calcaneoquartile joint
Lateral collateral
ligament (long p.)
Trochlea
of the talus
23
Tarsometatarsal joint

See key to the table on page 86

fig.22.14
Enlarged picture of the anterior view showing the position of the tarsal ligaments.

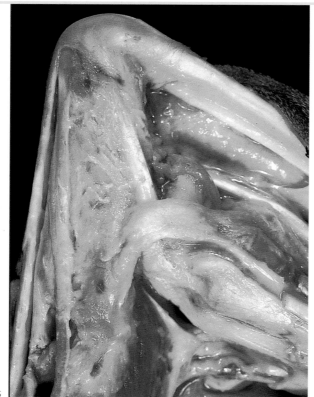

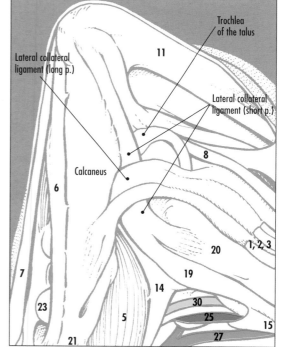

Trochlea
of the talus
Lateral collateral
ligament (long p.)
11
Lateral collateral
ligament (short p.)
8
Calcaneus
6
1, 2, 3
7
20
19
14
23
30
5
25
21
15
27

See key to the table on page 86

fig.22.15
Tarsal ligaments in hyperflexion.

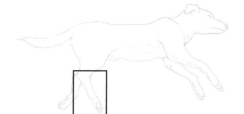

23

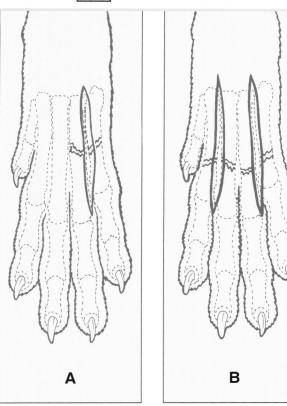

A

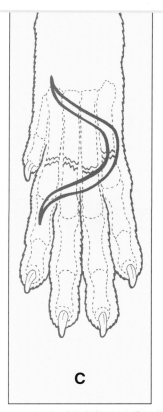

B

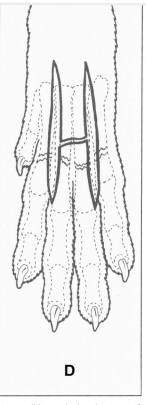

C

D

The same cutaneous incision used for the metacarpal bones is valid for the metatarsals. If only one metatarsal is involved, the incision will be made directly over it. If two are involved, the incision will be between them (A). If the four metatarsal bones are affected, different incisions are available (B, C, D).

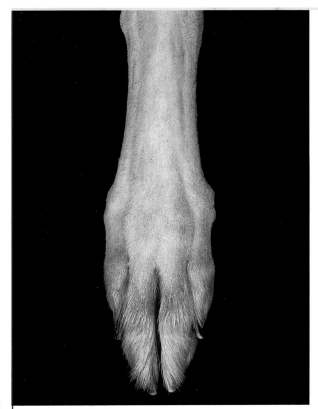

fig.23.1

The animal is in sternal recumbency. Dorsal view of the left pelvic paw.

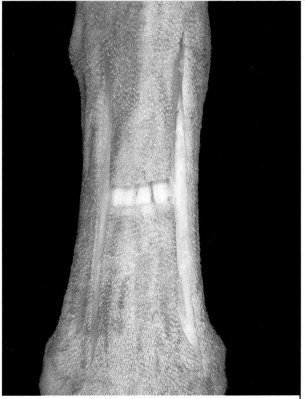

fig.23.2

The cutaneous incision to approach the four metatarsal bones is "H" shaped, with the centre (cross-bar) of the incision at the middle of the shaft of the metatarsals.

23

The dorsal common digital veins are close to the dorsal common digital arteries and nerves but due to their small size are difficult to identify.

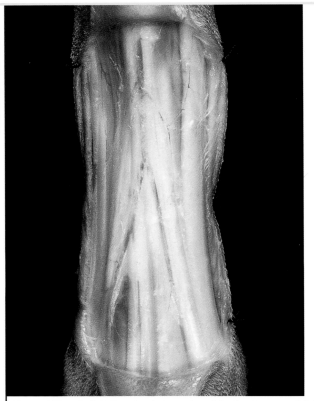

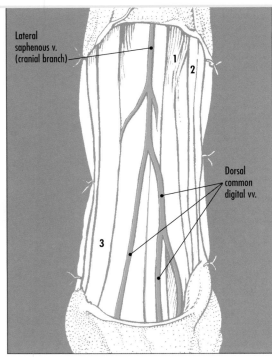

1 - Short digital extensor m. 2 - Tendon of the lateral digital extensor m. 3 - Metatarsal bone II.

fig.23.3

The cranial branch of the lateral saphenous vein and the dorsal common digital veins are dissected free from deeper structures. If the small neurovascular branches are accidentally cut during the approach, no clinical repercussions are encountered.

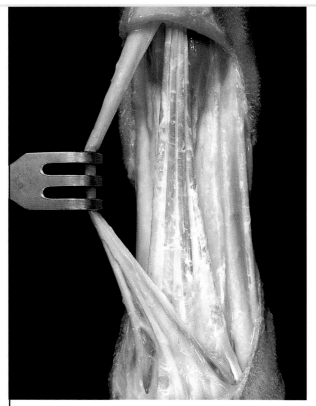

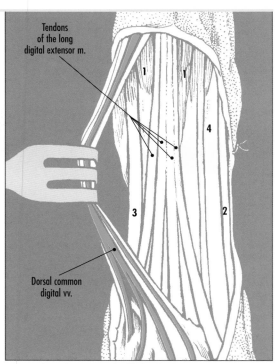

1 - Extensor digitorum brevis m. 2 - Tendon of the lateral digital extensor m. 3 - Metatarsal bone II.
4 - Metatarsal bone V.

fig.23.4

After medial retraction of the neurovascular structures, the four tendons of insertion of the long digital extensor muscle may be identified.

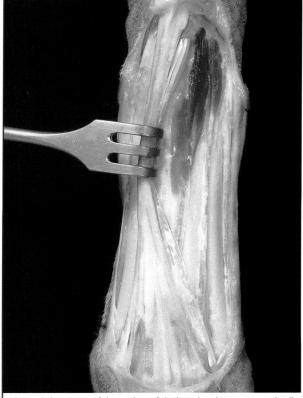

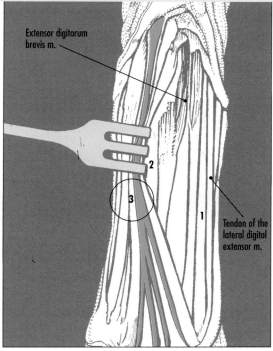

Extensor digitorum brevis m.

2

3

1

Tendon of the lateral digital extensor m.

1 - Metatarsal bone V **2** - Metatarsal bone III **3** - Dorsal common digital vv., tendons of the long digital extensor m.

fig.23.5

The medial retraction of the tendons of the long digital extensor muscle allows the visualisation of the bellies and tendons of the extensor digitorum brevis muscle.

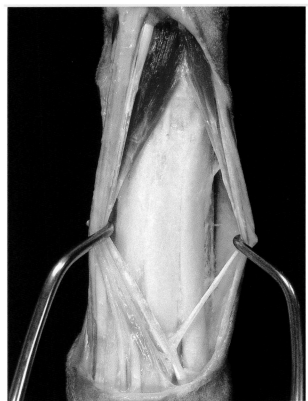

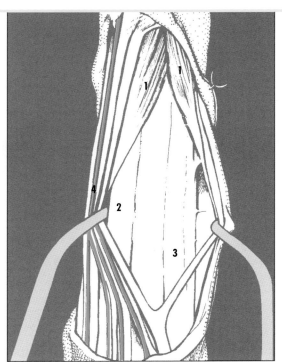

1

1

4

2

3

1 - Extensor digitorum brevis m. **2** - Metatarsal II **3** - Metatarsal V **4** - Dorsal common digital vv., tendons of long digital extensor and extensor digitorum brevis mm.

fig.23.6

The metatarsal bones II, III, IV and V are exposed by retracting laterally or medially the tendons of the extensor digitorum brevis muscle and the more superficial structures.

References

Piermattei DL (1993). An Atlas of Surgical Approaches to the Bones and Joints of the Dog and Cat. 3rd Ed. WB Saunders Co, Philadelphia.

Nomina Anatomica Veterinaria. (1994). 4th Ed. The World Association of Veterinary Anatomists. Zurich.

Evans EE (1993). Miller´s Anatomy of the Dog. 3rd Ed. WB Saunders Co, Philadelphia.

Brinker WO, Piermattei DL, Flo G (1997). Handbook of Small Animal Orthopedics and Fracture Treatment. 3rd Ed. WB Saunders Co, Philadelphia.